DENTAL SCIENCE, MATERIALS AND TECHNOLOGY

IMPLANTS IN CONTEMPORARY ORTHODONTICS

DENTAL SCIENCE, MATERIALS AND TECHNOLOGY

Additional books in this series can be found on Nova's website under the Series tab.

Additional e-books in this series can be found on Nova's website under the e-book tab.

DENTAL SCIENCE, MATERIALS AND TECHNOLOGY

IMPLANTS IN CONTEMPORARY ORTHODONTICS

DEVINDER PREET SINGH

NOVA BIOMEDICAL

New York

Library of Congress Cataloging-in-Publication Data

ISBN: 978-1-63484-302-7

Published by Nova Science Publishers, Inc. † New York

Contents

Preface		**vii**
Introduction		**1**
History		**3**
Chapter 1	Review of Literature	**5**
Chapter 2	Medical Evaluation of the Patient	**15**
Chapter 3	Radiologic Planning for Dental Implants	**17**
Chapter 4	Classification of Implants	**25**
Chapter 5	Materials Used for Implants	**31**
Chapter 6	Biocompatibility of Titanium Implants	**33**
Chapter 7	Implant Design Properties	**41**
Chapter 8	Factors Influencing Osseointegration	**45**
Chapter 9	Healing of Endosseous Implants	**51**
Chapter 10	Restorative Considerations in Combined Orthodontic Implant Therapy	**59**
Chapter 11	Experiments Regarding the Stability of Implant Materials	**63**
Chapter 12	Clinical Uses of Implants in Orthodontics	**65**
Chapter 13	Newer Implant Systems	**77**

Chapter 14 Implants and Distraction Osteogenesis **107**

Conclusion **117**

Bibliography **119**

About the Author **127**

Index **129**

Preface

Skeletal Anchorage System (SAS) involves the use of implants as a source of orthodontic anchorage. Implants are fast gaining popularity as their patient compliance expectation use is minimal. Anchorage can be both orthodontic as well as orthopedic. The orthopedic uses include maxillary expansion as well as maxillary protraction while orthodontic uses include intrusion, space closure and distalization. With the development of newer implants such as the micro-implants, the concept of absolute anchorage has been revolutionized as these implants are small, easily placed as well as removed, and require minimal healing period before loading.

It should be understood that the techniques presented are a vehicle by which a principle is demonstrated. The principle can be achieved by these as well as, perhaps, by other means. It is the principle that is important, the principle as defined within the limitation of our present-day understanding.

References are used where it is believed appropriate and within my ability to document sources of information. It has been my intent to give proper credit wherever possible. I believe the reference lists have scientific merit. While there is much that remains to be known about the practice of orthodontic implants, this text represents a continuing quest for the truth, and my interpretation of the present state of dentistry as a science and art. The future of implants in orthodontics is promising, as product developments in terms of minimal patient discomfort and reduced treatment time are continually occurring. I am immensely grateful to the Almighty God who showered me with his choicest blessings and enlightened me to carry out this project successfully. I wish to express my sincere gratitude to my parents, whose unforgettable sacrifices and choicest blessings provided me the opportunity to be educated enough to be in a position to write this current literature.

Devinder Preet Singh, BDS, MDS.

Introduction

As the glorious first century of organized orthodontics has passed and we have entered in next century, the sheer pace of technological advancement is awesome. If the history of all landmarks were to be drawn, the most recent would be the development of the Skeletal Anchorage System (SAS).

Skeletal Anchorage System (SAS) involves the use of implants as source of orthodontic anchorage. The pioneering studies on oral implants was done by LINKOW in 1967 [1] who is rightfully called the Father of Oral Implantology.

Implants are fast gaining popularity as with their use patient compliance expectation is minimal. Anchorage can be both orthodontic as well as orthopedic. The orthopedic uses include maxillary expansion as well as maxillary protraction while orthodontic include intrusion, space closure and distalization.

Now with the development of newer implants such as the micro-implants their use has been revolutionized as these implants are small, easily placed as well as removed and require minimal healing period before loading. The future of implants in orthodontics is promising as product developments in terms of minimal patient discomfort and reduced treatment time are continually occurring.

History

The origin of dental implants for replacing missing teeth began as early as the Greeks, Etruscans, and Egyptians. These civilizations employed different designs and materials ranging from jade to bone to metal. Some of the designs they used have evolved into the modern implants we see today.

Albucasis de Condue (936-1013) [2] attempted to use ox bone to replace missing teeth and this treatment was the first documented placement of implants. Towards the 18th century, *Pierre Fauchard* [2] and *John Hunter* [2] further documented tooth transplantation with conditions for it's success. In *1809 Maggiolo* [3] fabricated gold roots that were fixed to pivot teeth by means of a spring. These gold implants were placed into fresh extraction sites although not truly submerged into bone. The crowns were placed after healing had occurred around the implant. *Harris* [4] followed in *1887* with the implantation of a platinum post coated with lead. The post was shaped like a tooth root, and the lead was roughened for retention into the socket. *Bonwill* [5] in *1895*, used gold or iridium tubes implanted into bone to restore a single tooth or to support complete dentures. *Payne (1898)* [6], implanted a silver capsule as a foundation for a porcelain crown that was cemented several weeks later. In *1905 Scholl* [2] demonstrated a porcelain corrugated tooth implant. The implant was successful for two years and was anchored to adjacent teeth and fillings through the use of pins. In *1913 Greenfield* [7] introduced a hollow basket implant made from a meshwork of 24-gauge iridium-platinum wires soldered wit a 24-carat gold. This was used to support single implants, as well as fixed partial dentures using as many as eight implants. *Adams in 1937* [8] patented a submergible threaded cylindrical implant with a round bottom, smooth gingival collar, and a healing cap. In *1938, Strock* [9] placed a threaded vitallium implant which had a cone shaped head for the cementation of a jacket crown.

Shortly thereafter in *1982* in Toronto, *Branemark* [10] presented a work began fifteen years back and the principles of osseointegration were set forth.

Chapter 1

Review of Literature

Gainesforth et al. (1945) [11], conducted a study in which they used titanium screws for orthodontic anchorage in six dogs. These implants were inserted in the ramus area and immediately attached to a device designed to retract the maxillary cuspids. They found that all the screws are lost within 16-31 days.

Alan J. Sherman (1978) [12], studied the movement of vitreous carbon implants under the stress of a classic orthodontic force. The implants were inserted into the extraction sites of the mandibular third premolars in dogs. The implants were allowed to heal for 70 days before being loaded with 175 gms of force. After 7 weeks they observed that of the original six implant sites, two of the implant sites were firm, functional and considered to be successful. A third implant had some mobility; it functioned, but the degree of success was questionable. The gross measurements of the interdental space mesial and distal to the implants never varied more than 0.5 mm from the original measurements.

John R. Smith (1979) [13], conducted a study in which aluminium oxide implants coated with bio-glass were placed bilaterally in the mandibular first molar region of three male *Macaca mulatta* monkeys. A lingual arch appliance with continuous lingual force was directed to the endosteal implants. Fusion of the implants to the surrounding bone was achieved in five of the six implants and remained intact throughout loading periods of 2,5 and 9 weeks in five of the six implants using 425 to 925 grams of force. The implant-bone union offered a barrier to downward migration of epithelium and inflammation.

Guyman et al. (1980) [14], conducted a study in which they ankylosed the maxillary permanent lateral incisors of three rhesus monkeys by replantation and splinting technique. A 1 pound expansion force was applied to the ankylosed teeth for 5-15 weeks. They observed that skeletal expansion of the maxilla was achieved without concomitant buccal tipping of the abutment teeth. Osteoid tissue was deposited on localized areas of the resorbed cementum and dentin of the ankylosed teeth.

Gray et al. (1983) [15], conducted a study to test the abilities of Bio-glass coated and vitallium small cylindrical endosseous implants to resist movement when loaded with constant forces of orthodontic magnitudes. These were implanted in the femurs of 12 rabbits. After a 28 day healing period, these implants were loaded with forces of 60 gms, 120 gms and 180 gms. Analysis of implant movement after 28 days revealed that no statistically significant movement occurred at any of the three force levels for either type of implant.

Eugene Roberts et al. (1984) [16], conducted a study in which they inserted pure titanium screw implants with an acid etched surface into the femurs of 3-6 month old rabbits. After 6-12 weeks of healing, a 100 gm load was applied for 4-8 weeks by stretching a stainless steel spring between the implants. They found that all but one of twenty loaded implants remained rigid and immediate loading of four pairs of implants resulted in spontaneous spiral type (torsional) fractures of the femur within 1 week.

The results indicated that – *1.* Relatively simple and inexpensive titanium implants develop a rigid osseous interface. *2.* 6 weeks is an adequate healing period, prior to loading, to attain rigid stability and avoid spontaneous fracture. *3.* Continuously loaded implants remained stable within the bone. *4.* Bone formation is observed on periosteal surfaces subjected to concave flexure (compression). *5.* Cancellous type bone orients perpendicularly between loaded implants, apparently corresponding to lines of stress. *6.* New secondary osteons are propagated at or near the surface of loaded implants. The remodeling (turnover) cycle for rabbit compact bone is about 6 weeks. *7.* Endosseous implants have potential as a source of firm osseous anchorage for orthodontics and dentofacial orthopedics.

Smalley et al. (1988) [17], conducted a study in which they placed titanium implants surgically into the maxillary, zygomatic, frontal, occipital & orbital bones of four pigtail monkeys. Using an external protraction device attached to the orbital and occipital implants, a constant force of 600 gms per side was applied to the maxillary or zygomatic bones for 12-18 weeks. They demonstrated a 12 mm widening of the zygomaticomaxillary suture and 16 mm of the zygomaticotemporal sutures, a change from Class I to Class II dental relationship and increase in overjet of 5-7mm. The facial implants remained immobile throughout the experiment.

Turley et al. (1988) [18], conducted a study in six young adult mongrel dogs to investigate the use of titanium endosseous implants as anchors for orthodontic tooth movement and to examine the stability of these implants when placed in nontraditional sites such as the mandibular lingual plate and the palate intraorally, and the zygoma and temporal bone extraorally. They found that out of a total of 42 implants which were placed, 24 remained stable. Of these 24 implants, 8 received activation. The remainder served as unloaded controls.

Eugene Roberts et al. (1989) [19], conducted a study on dog mandibles and found that clinical rigidity was achieved by 94% of the titanium implants. All loaded implants remained rigid. Inadvertent impingement on the periodontal ligament and roots of adjacent teeth are uneventful. They also observed that implants with teeth was uneventful. They also observed that implants with less than 10% of the endosseous interface in direct contact with bone successfully resisted a continuous load of 3 N (>300 gms) for 13 weeks.

Eugene Roberts et al. (1989) [20], conducted a study in five adult patients in which retromolar dental implants served as anchorage to close first molar extraction sites. Rates of unidirectional space closure for mandibular second molars were assessed with periapical radiographs superimposed on anatomical landmarks and retromolar anchorage implants. They concluded that sustained orthodontic translation is a physiological manifestation of bone modeling and remodeling throughout the adjacent alveolar process and the rate of mandibular molar translation is inversely related to the apparent radiographic density of the resisting alveolar bone.

Block and Hoffman (1995) [21], conducted a dog study to determine the ability of the onplant, once biointegrated to bone, to remain stable when subjected to orthodontic forces. Four mongrel dogs were used.

In each dog two onplants were placed onto the palate. In addition, one onplant was placed over the lateral ramus for mechanical testing in two dogs. A spring was placed and attached to the ball abutment within the onplant. The spring was activated between the tooth and the abutment to exert 11 ounces of force. The springs were checked weekly and reactivated when needed. All the dogs were killed after 5 months.

They found that the onplants did not move in relation to the incisors or the molars. However, the premolar attached to the onplant moved toward the onplant in each animal. At the conclusion of the study, one tooth moved 4 mm and the other two teeth had moved 8 mm. The soft tissue around the onplant was normal in appearance, with slight inflammation consistent with plaque accumulation.

Block and Hoffman (1995) [21], conducted a monkey study to simulate an intended use of the onplant to stabilize molars during retraction of the anterior dentition to mimic a situation commonly encountered in clinical orthodontics. Five monkeys were used in the study. One monkey served as a control, and the remaining four had one onplant placed in the middle of the palate opposite the maxillary second molar. Two onplants had sharp 90° peripheral edges and two had tapered edges. After 12 weeks for healing, the onplants were exposed and the abutments placed. At the time of onplant placement, the monkeys' first and second maxillary premolars were extracted bilaterally, creating space between the maxillary first molars and the canines. Bilateral stainless steel springs were stretched from the canines to the first molars. They exerted a 250 gm reciprocal force between the first molars and the canines. The springs were calibrated weekly to keep the forces as constant as possible. The monkeys were killed after 6 months. They found that the anchored molars moved an average of 1. 2 ± 0.2 mm toward the central incisors. The non-anchored molars moved an average of 4.1 ± 1.4 mm toward the central incisors ($p < 0.01$). The canines on the anchored side moved an average of 1.9 ± 0.6 mm away from the central incisors, and the canines on the non-anchored side moved an average of 1.9 ± 0.7 mm away from the central incisors ($p > 0.01$).

Southard et al. (1995) [22], conducted a study to compare the intrusion anchorage potential of teeth to osseointegrated titanium implants. Titanium implants were surgically placed unilaterally in a healed mandibular fourth premolar extraction site in eight adult mongrel dogs. The implants were surgically uncovered 3 months later and second stage abutments with soldered edgewise brackets secured. Edgewise brackets were also placed on the ipsilateral third premolars and on the contralateral third and fourth premolars. Segmental edgewise arch wires were placed between the implant and the third premolar and between the contralateral third and fourth premolars. Intrusion arch wire bends (v-bends) just mesial to the implant and the fourth premolar brackets were adjusted to apply a 50 to 60 gm intrusive force to the third premolars, bilaterally. Seven weeks later this force was increased to approximately 100 gm. Force levels were monitored biweekly for a total period of 16 weeks. Superimposition of initial and final periapical radiographs with bone markers demonstrated that for each dog the implant remained immobile and the third premolar on the implant anchor side was intruded in a curved path. On the contralateral side of the arch the dental anchor (fourth premolar) underwent an adverse reactive tip-back movement, and the third premolar was not intruded. They concluded that rigid endosseous implants are superior to dental anchorage for orthodontic intrusion of teeth and offer a potential means to intrude anterior teeth in adult patients with missing posterior teeth.

Parr et al. (1997) [23], conducted a study in which they placed two flanged titanium implants on either side of the midnasal suture of 18 New Zealand white rabbits. One experimental group was loaded at 1N and the other at 3N. All rabbits were euthanized after 12 weeks of loading. They observed that the distance between the implants increased significantly in the loaded groups compared with the control, and was significantly higher in the 3 N than in the 1 N group. They also observed that relatively low loads (1 or 3 N) applied to rigidly integrated endosseous implants across an unfused suture are satisfactory for achieving expansion under the conditions of the study.

Nergiz et al. (1998) [24], studied the functional and morphologic reactions of peri-implant bone surrounding screw implants (Bonefit) in three dogs by loading the implants with continuous forces of 2 N (about 204 gm) and 5 N (about 510 gm). Eight implants were inserted to an endosseous length of 12 mm and placed about 10 mm apart in the region of the lower premolars. The fixtures healed in a closed environment for 12 weeks, after which they were uncovered and loaded with abutments and orthodontic devices to produce horizontal distraction with a force of 2 N (about 204 gm) for 12 weeks. Subsequently they were loaded with 5 N (about 510 gm) for another 24 weeks. The distance between and the mobility of the implants were determined before and after each phase of experimental loading. Fixtures of the same type that were osseointegrated and not exposed, or osseointegrated and loaded by mastication, were used as a control. Animals were euthanized and specimens sectioned. The result was that continuously loaded implants showed no significant displacement for any force level. The mobility of the fixtures increased slightly by about 1 Periotestvalue (PTV) at the end of the experiment. Histologic and morphometric evaluation indicated compaction of bone as a result of loading. Osseointegrated implants have potential as a firm osseous anchorage for orthodontic treatment and can resist continuous horizontal forces of at least 5 N (about 510 gm) during a period of several months.

De Pauw et al. (1999) [25], conducted an animal study to investigate the stability of osseointegrated fixtures when used as anchorage for orthopaedic traction with extreme force magnitude. Three Branemark fixtures were placed in the left zygomatic arch and three in the right of five adult dogs. An orthopedic nonaxial force of 5 N was applied using an intraoral coil system. After 2 months of continuous loading, all loaded implants were immobile. Significant marginal bone loss at the abutment fixture interface (< 1mm) was observed around each loaded fixture implant. Bone remodeling was significantly more pronounced at the tension side of the implants, irrespective of fixture length. Radiographical and histological analyses showed bone with normal trabecular pattern around the implants.

Wehrbein et al. (1999) [26], conducted a clinical and radiological study to estimate the necessary palatal bone support required for orthodontic implant anchorage. Twelve patients (six male and six female) aged 15-39 years received a Straumann Orthosystem implant in the mid-sagittal palatal area for achieving maximum anchorage in the maxilla during orthodontic treatment. The bone thickness in the implantation site was verified by probing during the implantation of the implant and then compared with the thickness as measured on the lateral cephalogram.

They found that vertical bone support is atleast 2mm higher than apparent on the cephalogram. Thus, they concluded that the mid-sagittal area of the palate lends sufficient bony support for the implantation of small implants (4-6 mm endosseous length, diameter 3.3 mm).

Wehrbein et al. (1999) [26], conducted a prospective study to evaluate the anchorage capacity of palatally inserted Orthosystem implants for anchorage reinforcement of posterior teeth. The sample consisted of 9 dental Class II patients (age 15 to 35 years) whose treatment plan included extraction of the maxillary first premolars. Each of the patients received 1 implant inserted into the center of the anterior palate. After a mean unloaded implant healing period of 3 months, transpalatal bars were inserted to connect the posterior teeth to the implant. Retraction of the canines and incisors was accomplished without the use of compliance-dependent headgear or Class II elastics. The degree of anchorage loss as well as the amount of canine and incisor retraction were evaluated by measurements of the casts and lateral cephalograms. They found that the mean anchorage loss was 0.7 mm on the right side and 1.1 mm on the left ($P < .05$). The right and left canines were retracted 6.6 and 6.4 mm, respectively, and the mean overjet reduction was 6.2 mm.

Majzoub et al. (1999) [27], conducted a study to evaluate the effect of early orthodontic loading on the stability and bone implant interface of titanium implants in a rabbit model. Twenty- four short threaded fixtures were inserted into the calvarial mid-sagittal suture of 10 rabbits. Two weeks following insertion, 20 implants (test group) were subjected to continuous distalization forces 150 gram for a period of 8 weeks. The remaining four implants (control group) were left unloaded for the same follow-up interval. They found that clinically all implants except one test fixture were stable, and exhibited no mobility or displacement throughout the experimental loading period. Morphometrically, a bone to implant contact of 76.00 ± 18.73% was found on the test pressure sides and 75.00 ± 11.54% at the test tension sides and 69.00 ± 15.55% on the control unloaded surfaces. They concluded that short endosseous implants can be used as anchoring units for orthodontic tooth movement early in the post-insertion healing period.

Shigeru Saito et al. (2000) [28], conducted a study to determine the anchorage potential of titanium implants (Brånemark; 3.75, 7mm) with the use of a sectional arch wire technique for orthodontic mesiodistal tooth movement, as assessed by the osseointegration of implants and tooth movement. Two implants were surgically placed in healed mandibular extraction sites of the second and third premolars on each side in 4 adult male beagle dogs. They observed that not only was there no statistical difference in the percent of peri-implant bone volume between the loaded and unloaded sides, but there was also no statistical difference between the compression and tension sides in both loaded and unloaded implants, which suggests that the implants maintained rigid osseointegration. Thus, the study demonstrated that endosseous titanium implants can function as anchors for long-term orthodontic mesiodistal movement.

Daimaruya et al. (2001) [29], conducted a study to verify the effect of molar intrusion on the neurovascular bundle, the level of osseointegration of bone screws, and root resorption. The results of this study showed mandibular molars were intruded 3.4 mm on the average over 7 months in dogs. The miniplates were well stabilized with osseointegrated bone screws and the peri-implant soft tissues showed slight inflammatory changes. Neither nerves nor blood vessels were damaged. Root resorption was observed but was repaired with new cementum. They concluded that the Skeletal Anchorage System (SAS) utilizing transmucosal titanium miniplates as an immovable orthodontic anchorage could provide a new modality for molar intrusions without serious iatrogenic problems.

Ohmae et al. (2001) [30], conducted a study to determine the anchorage potential of the titanium mini-implant for orthodontic intrusion of the mandibular posterior teeth. Six mini-implants were surgically placed around the mandibular third premolars on each side in 3 adult male beagle dogs. In 6 weeks, an intrusive force (150 g) was applied between the interradicular implants on the buccal and the lingual sites by closed coil springs run across the crowns of the third premolars. After 12 to 18 weeks of orthodontic intrusion, the animals were killed and their mandibles were dissected and prepared for histologic and fluorescent observation. They found that the mandibular third premolars intruded 4.5 mm, on average, after 12 to 18 weeks of orthodontic force application, with mild root resorption at the furcation area as well as the root apex. All the mini-implants remained stable during orthodontic tooth movement without any mobility or displacement. The morphometrical findings indicated that the calcification of the periimplant bone on the loaded implants was equal to or slightly greater than those of the controls. In addition, 6 of the 36 mini-implants were removed after tooth movement, and all of them were easily removed with a screwdriver.

Thilander et al. (2001) [31], conducted a study to evaluate the long term use of implants installed in different areas in adolescents. The sample consisted of 18 subjects with missing teeth (congenital absence or trauma). The patients were between the age group of 13-17 years and of different skeletal maturation. In all subjects the existing permanent teeth were fully erupted. In 15 patients 29 single implants were installed to replace premolars, canines and upper incisors. In three patients with extensive aplasia, 18 implants were placed in various regions. The patients were followed during a 10 year period, the first four years annually, and then every second year. Photographs, study casts, peri-apical radiographs, lateral cephalograms and body height measurements were recorded at each control. They concluded that dental implants are a good treatment option for replacing missing teeth in adolescence. However, different problems are related to the premolar and the incisor regions, which have to be considered in the total treatment planning.

Gedrange et al. (2003) [32], conducted a finite element study with three types of endosseous implants (all 9 mm in length and 3.3 mm in diameter, made of titanium). Type 1 was a simple, cylinder-shaped implant; type 2 a cylinder-shaped implant with a superperiosteal step; and type 3 a cylinder-shaped implant, subperiosteally threaded, with a superperiosteal step. The load on the implant was investigated under three conditions of bite and orthodontic forces from 0.01 to 100 N (vertically, horizontally, and diagonally). They concluded that vertical loading caused bone deformation of more than 600 μeps at the simple implant. The largest deformations at this load were found in the trabecular bone with all three implant geometries. However, trabecular bone deformation was reduced by a superperiosteal step. Horizontal loading of the implants shifted the deformation from the trabecular to the cortical bone. Furthermore, a large deformation was measured at the transition from cortical to trabecular bone. The smallest deformations (less than 300 μeps) were found for implants with a superperiosteal step and diagonal loading (type 2). The use of threads provided no improvement in loading capacity.

Erverdi et al. (2004) [33], conducted a study to assess the effectiveness of skeletal anchorage in the zygomatic buttress region for intrusion of maxillary posterior teeth, to correct open bite malocclusion and to evaluate the usage of titanium miniplates for orthodontic anchorage. Titanium miniplates were fixed bilaterally to the zygomatic buttress area and a force was applied bilaterally with 9mm Ni-Ti coil springs between the vertical extension of the mini-plate and the first molar buccal tube in ten patients 17 to 23 years old, characterized with an anterior open bite and excessively maxillary posterior growth. They concluded that 3.7mm of anterior open bite was corrected by 2.6mm maxillary molar intrusion, 1.1mm maxillary and mandibular incisor extrusion, 3.1° clockwise rotation of the maxillary occlusal plane and 1.7° counterclockwise rotation of the mandible. Thus, the zygomatic area was found to be a useful anchorage site for intrusion of the molars in a short period of time.

Trisi et al. (2004) [34], conducted a clinical, radiographic and histologic evaluation of the tissue surrounding SLA (sandblasted and acid etched) implants, placed in the maxilla of 3 dogs and mandible of 5 dogs after a 12 week healing period after extraction. The implants were loaded with a continuous and constant force for 52 weeks, after a healing period of 6 weeks, after implant insertion. Abutments were attached to the 6 test implants (2 in the maxilla, 4 in the mandible). Superelastic nickel-titanium coil springs were activated between the SLA implants and the canines, producing a force of 200g (2N). Two unloaded implants (1 in the maxilla, 1 in the mandible) served as controls. They observed that the corticalization of bone trabeculae was thicker at the loaded than the unloaded implants as well as new bone formation was superior at the level of the crest in the test implants. The mean bone-implant contact values of the test implants for the maxilla and mandible were 40.23% and 49.33% respectively. In the control implants, the bone-implant contact value was 67.91% for the maxilla and 49.23% for the mandible. Thus they concluded that SLA implants can be used as an anchorage unit with confidence in spite of a short healing period and a prolonged force application.

Sugawara et al. (2004) [35], conducted a study to evaluate the treatment and post-treatment changes during and after distalization of 29 mandibular molars with SAS (skeletal anchorage system) in 15 adult patients (12 women and 3 men). The amount of distalization and relapse and the type of tooth movement were analyzed with cephalometric radiographs and dental casts. They observed that the average amount of distalization of the mandibular first molars was 3.5 mm at the crown level and 1.8mm at the root level. The average amount of relapse was 0.3 mm at both the crown and root apex levels. Of 29 mandibular molars, 9 were tipped back, and others were translated distally in accordance with the established treatment goals. They concluded that SAS is a viable modality to move mandibular molars for distally correcting anterior crossbites, malocclusions characterized by mandibular anterior crowding, and dental asymmetries.

Oyonarte et al. (2005) [36], conducted a study to compare the bone response to orthodontic loading around 2 different types of osseointegrated implants (porous surfaced and machine threaded) to determine their suitability for orthodontic anchorage. Five beagle dogs each received 3 implants of each design in contralateral mandibular locations. After a 6 week initial healing period, abutments were placed and, 1week later, the 2 mesial implants on each side were orthodontically loaded for 22 weeks. Light microscopy and back-scattered scanning electron microscopy were used to compare responses around the 2 implant designs. They observed that porous-surfaced implants had a higher marginal bone levels and less relative implant displacement than machine-threaded implants. Significant differences in peri-implant bone remodeling and bone formation in response to controlled orthodontic loading were also observed in the 2 implant designs. They thus, concluded that short porous surfaced implants might be more effective for orthodontic applications than machine-threaded implants.

Chapter 2

Medical Evaluation of the Patient

Cardiovascular Assessment

Myocardial infarction is the most common cause of perioperative death in patients undergoing a surgical procedure. Other cardiovascular diseases, such as hypertension, congestive heart failure, valvular heart disease, and rhythm and conduction disturbances, are also commonly encountered.

Hypertension

Assessment of the patient with hypertension should focus on the detection of associated cardiac risk factors from the history and cursory examination. The history should focus on the duration of the patient's hypertension and specific treatment the patient is receiving and its effectiveness. The examination should include careful measurement of the blood pressure with a cuff of appropriate size.

Coronary Artery Disease

The preoperative evaluation of the patient with known or suspected coronary artery disease depends on the presence of residual myocardial ischemia, ventricular irritability and overall ventricular function.

Cigarette Smoking and Alcohol Abuse

Consideration should be given to the effects of cigarette smoke on surgical healing as well as to its better-know effects on the human body. Although no conclusive evidence exists to guide in the length of abstinence from smoking, many surgeons empirically ask their patients to refrain from smoking for 10 days before surgery and for 3 weeks after surgery.

The most notable problems in alcoholics for any proposed implant surgery include liver dysfunction, coagulopathies, abnormal white cell function, anemia, cardiac disorders, neurologic disorders, and alcohol withdrawal. The key to management is to obtain an accurate and thorough history from patients and to investigate any suspected alcohol abuse with laboratory studies so potential problems can be identified preoperatively.

Chapter 3

Radiologic Planning for Dental Implants

The first step in formulating a treatment plan for dental rehabilitation using implants must be determination of sufficient bone quantity and quality to support the implants. The choice of radiologic technique appropriate for a given patient depends on a number of factors, including the type of restoration and implants to be used, the position of the remaining dentition and the extent to which bone quality or quantity is in question.

Radiologic Methods

1. Periapical Radiographs

Periapical radiographs reveal the location of roots, either from teeth adjacent to the proposed implant site or from teeth that have been lost or extracted without removal of the entire root. They can also reveal the presence of other foreign bodies, such as stainless steel ligatures, bone plates, or screws that might interfere with the placement or osseointegration of an implant. If the maxillary central incisor area is being considered for an implant, Periapical radiographs can show the size and location of the incisive canal, which must be avoided because the epithelium within the canal may prevent osseointegration by enveloping the implant. Periapical radiographs are most valuable in monitoring crestal bone maintenance after implants are placed, particularly with superimposed millimeter grid marking.

Advantages

- They are available in most dental offices.
- All dentists are thoroughly trained to read the resulting radiographs.

Disadvantages

- Angulation distortion is present.
- Determination of actual ridge height is difficult because periapical radiographs do not have one-to-one correspondence with regard to size.

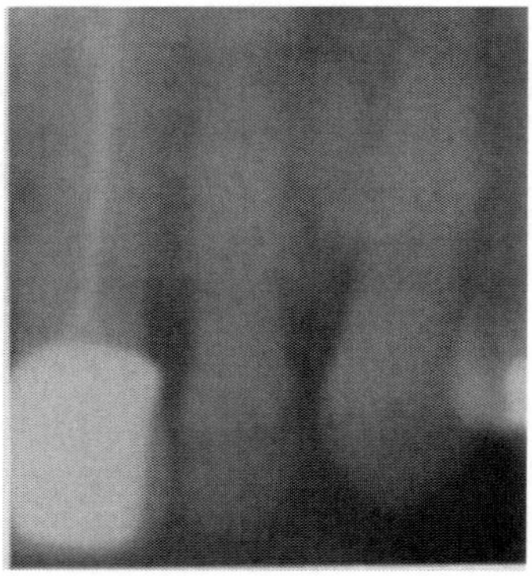

Figure 1. Periapical Radiograph.

2. Panoramic Radiographs

The most commonly used radiologic technique for preoperative planning is the panoramic radiograph, because it enables the dentist to visualize the presence or absence of dentition or other implants in both arches. It is also a useful screen for osseous disorders such as residual cysts.

Bone height in the mandible can be accurately assessed using a marker of a known size placed directly on the mucosa when the panoramic radiograph is obtained. For example, if the markers actually have a diameter of 5mm; however, on the panoramic film they measure 6 mm - a 20% distortion. Therefore, although the panoramic radiograph shows 22 mm of bone above the inferior alveolar canal in the lower left first molar area, only 18.3 mm is actually available; in the lower right first molar area, 24mm of bone is measurable above the inferior alveolar canal, but only 20mm of bone is actually available.

A panoramic radiograph can indicate the anterio-posterior location of the mental foramen relative to the proposed implant site. As long as the proposed implant site is 3mm or more anterior to the mental foramen, a long endosteal implant that engages the inferior cortical bone of the mandible can be used. If the mental foramina are at the surface of the resorbed mandible, the incision for osseous exposure should be placed toward the lingual aspect of the alveolar process to avoid damaging the mental nerve as the mandibular symphysis is exposed.

Panoramic radiographs provide definitive information regarding the height of the alveolar bone; they do not, however, provide information about the width of bone. Because the maxillary mucosa is of variable thickness, accurate width prediction is problematic. Cross-sectional imaging should be used to confirm anticipated maxillary bone volume before placement of dental implants. When inadequate maxillary bone is available, the patient should be advised of various bone augmentation techniques to restore maxillary bone volume, combined with endosteal implants.

Panoramic radiographs do not provide sufficient diagnostic information about the size and shape of the maxillary sinuses. The concave floor of the sinus results in variable dimensions of the alveolar process anteroposteriorly as well as mediolaterally. Conventional panoramic radiographs show the bone height that is present within the focal trough of the panograph. The paucity of diagnostic information relative to the floor of the maxillary sinus is appreciated when one compares the conventional panograph to the three-dimensional image provided by the special dental processing software that is used to process CT images.

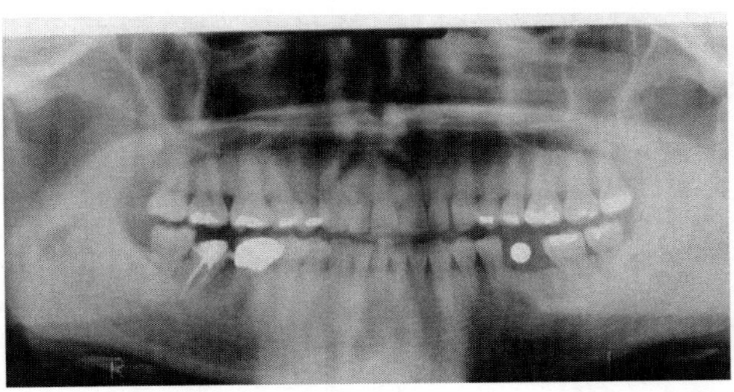

Figure 2. Panoramic Radiograph.

Advantages of panoramic radiographs are that both arches are present on one film, most dental offices are equipped and staffed to obtained panoramic radiographs, and all dentists are thoroughly trained to read the panoramic radiographs.

Disadvantages include lack of width determination of the alveolar process and magnification of structures.

3. Lateral Cephalometric Radiographs

Lateral cephalometric radiographs provide an exact image of the occlusal relationship between the arches and possible skeletal abnormalities. This relationship is important in determining the force that will be applied to any implant-borne restoration. When class I occlusion is not achievable, increased anterior maxillary or mandibular occlusal loading may develop. If the patient's age, general health, or reluctance to undergo orthognathic surgery prevents orthodontic or surgical correction of the skeletal abnormality, the abnormal concentration of forces generated by the alignment of the jaws must be considered when determining the number and size of the implants to support any dental restoration.

For patients who are edentulous in either or both arches, the lateral cephalometric radiograph allows the dentist to evaluate both the soft tissue profile and the relationship between the two arches. After a trial prosthesis is fabricated and coated with radiopaque material, a second cephalometric radiograph can be taken to determine the relationship of the proposed dental restoration to the residual osseous structure and to demonstrate aesthetics from the facial soft tissue profile generated by the proposed restoration.

The lateral cephalometric radiograph's one-to-one imaging of the buccal and lingual cortical heights of the mandibular symphysis allows the dentist to determine precisely the appropriate length and inclination of implants to be placed.

Advantages

- Availability from oral and maxillofacial surgeons and orthodontists.
- One-to-one images, and profile prediction.

Disadvantages

- The radiographs are not available in general dental offices,
- They provide information about the alveolar processes only relative to the midsagittal plane.

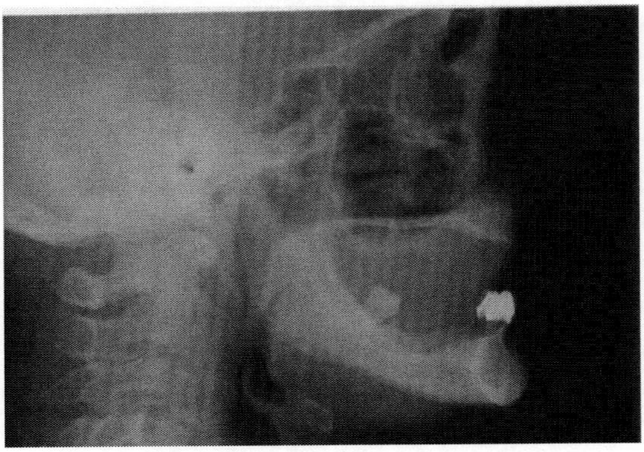

Figure 3. Lateral Cephalogram.

4. Conventional Tomograms

Conventional tomograms provide cross-sectional images that give the dentist precise information about bone volume and the location of vital structures when combined with markets of known size. When tomograms are ordered, communication between the dentist and the radiologist is of utmost importance because the dentist must precisely identify the specific area to be imaged. The dentist must also provide the radiologist with a radiologic marker of known dimension to be placed on the alveolar process in the plane of the tomogram. The advantage of conventional tomograms is reduction of radiation and cost compared with CT.

When radiographs of proposed sites for implant placement reveal inadequate bone volume, the dentist may request images of additional sites. Therefore, although a conventional tomogram results in less radiation exposure for the patient than a CT image, this advantage is diminished when multiple prospective implant sites are to be imaged. Many radiographers no longer maintain conventional tomographic equipment because CT has become the state of the art in tomography.

5. Computed Tomography

Since 1972, when the first computerized scanner converter x-ray pictures into digital signals, major changes in images have occurred. First CT used computer technology to offer images with dramatically enhanced detail. Conventional diagnostic radiographic techniques provide images with fewer than 30 variations of gray, whereas contemporary CT techniques generate images with more than 200 shades of gray. The increased CT gray scale shows subtle variations in tissue density that are not discernible with conventional radiology.

Second, special dental processing software programs capable of further enhancing the CT image to show three-dimensional images and one-to-one correspondence were introduced in 1987. These programs provide panoramic and cross-sectional images in addition to three-dimensional images of either the maxilla or the mandible. The dentist usually studies the three-dimensional images to gain an overview of the area being considered for implants, especially the contour of the bone being considered for implantation. Next the dentist studies the panographic views to develop an overall plan for each arch. The panographic images serves as a convenient image for patient counselling. Once the overall plan for each arch has been developed, the dentist uses the cross-sectional images, which include cross references to the panographic images, to determine the width and height of bone at the specific sites selected for individual implants. Knowing the precise height from the alveolar ridge to adjacent vital structures, such as the nasal floor or the inferior alveolar canal, allows the dentist to select the longest implant that will not violate any adjacent vital structure.

Two companies currently market software capable of providing three-dimensional images for dental implant planning. Software from 3D/Dental (Columbia Scientific, Inc, Columbia, MD) provides life-sized (one-to-one) panoramic and cross-sectional images as well as three-dimensional images, and the software from Dent/a/Scan (General Electric Co, Milwaukee, WI) provides a scale that the surgeon can use to convert measurements on the images accurately to actual size.

A computed tomographic appliance may be used both to facilitate patient positioning during the scanning process and to simplify correlation of the images at the time of implant placement. The appliance consists of a clear acrylic surgical guide that is modified by placement of a gutta percha line parallel to the proposed occlusal plane and gutta percha lines in the midbuccal facing and central fossa of each tooth that is a propose implant site. The CT technician uses the occlusal plan marker to ensure that the patient is in the proper position on the scanning Gantry before starting the actual scanning process. The surgeon and restorative dentists then modify the appliance after they review the scan so that the precise area selected on the scan is the area prepared for implant placement.

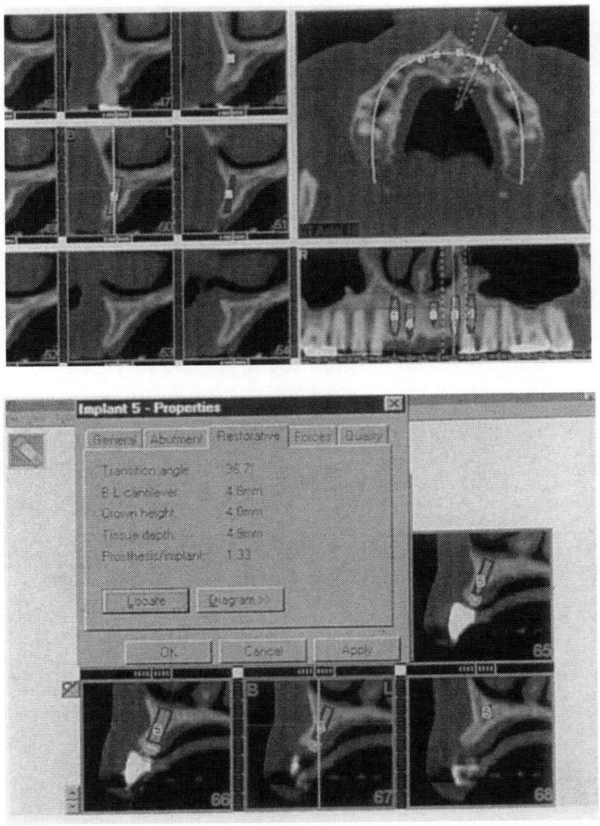

Figure 4. Computed Tomography Images.

SIM/PLANT (Columbia Scientific, Inc, Columbia, MD), an interactive dental implant software package that allows dentists to view and manipulate processed CT images on their office computers, became available in 1993. With SIM/PLANT for Window (Microsoft Corp, Redmond, WA), dentists can visualize vital structures and judge bone quantity and quantity using the life-size panoramic, cross-sectional, and transaxial images produced by CT that are processed on Columbia Scientific's Image Master-101 using IM/PLANT software. In addition to using the images to judge bone quality and quantity, dentists can use SIM/PLANT software to superimpose images of actual-size implants on theCT images for treatment planning and presentation purposes.

The advantage of CT is one-to-one imaging with unsurpassed detail relative to all potential implant sites within either the maxilla or the mandible. Disadvantages are that an appointment is necessary at a special facility with the appropriate CT scanner, images are more expensive than routine films, the patient is exposed to more radiation than with other radiologic techniques, and the dentist must be trained to read the resulting images.

6. Magnetic Resonance Imaging

The physical principle, or effect, that forms the basis of MRI is the interaction of nuclei, which have a non-zero magnetic moment with a magnetic field. Radiofrequency coils generate a magnetic field that is used to excite the nuclei and detect the signal. Similar to all digital images, magnetic resonance images are displayed via an image processor on a cathode-ray tube.

Tissues with relatively high water content is more precisely imaged with MRI technology than those tissues with relatively low moisture content. At present, bone imaging is not as detailed with MRI as it is with CT. MRI technology is not presently used in assessing the quantity and quality of bone that may be available for placement of dental implants.

Chapter 4

Classification of Implants

According to Block and Kent [9] implants may be classified as:

- Based on the location.
- Based on the configuration design.
- Based on the material.
- According to the surface texture.
- According to the mode of placement.

Location

Based on the location, implants may be (1) Subperiosteal (2) Transosseous (3) Endosseous implants.

1. Subperiosteal Implants - In this type implant body lies over the bony ridge. Even though it has the longest history of clinical trials, a decreased long term success rate probably due to the fact that the chances of getting dislodged are high. Also this complex design requires precise casting procedure. Because there is often not enough bone in which to place an endosteal implant, dentists turned to placing implants on and around bone rather than in it in the form of subperiosteal implants. In *1943, Dahl* [37] placed metal structures on the mandible and maxilla with four projecting posts. *Goldberg* and *Gershkoff* [38] made an impression taken of the mucosa covering the edentulous ridge. On the model produced from this impression they generated a multifenestrated narrow cobalt-chrome-molybdenum casting with four abutments that had little bone

coverage and a fit that was reasonably accurate [39]. The two-stage technique was refined by several clinicians [40-45]. Subsequently a series of modifications were made in the implant design [39]. A three dimensional replica of the mandible can now be developed from CT images, making it no longer mandatory to carry out extensive surgical dissection for a direct bone impression [46]. CT-generated CAD-CAM models, however, are not as precise as those obtained from a direct bone impression [47], and many surgeons still use the direct technique.

2. Transosseous Implants:-In this type the implant body penetrates the bone completely. They have a good success rate but are not widely used because of possible damage to the intrabony structures like nerves and blood vessels. In *1975, Small* [48-50] introduced the transosseous mandibular staple bone plate, a reconstructive device placed through a submental incision and attached to the mandible with multiple fixation and two transosseous screws to support a full arch prosthesis.Current application of this device has been limited to the mandible only. Other transosseous implants of historical and practical importance are the single transosseous implant of *Cranin* [51] and the transmandibular implant of *Bosker* [52].

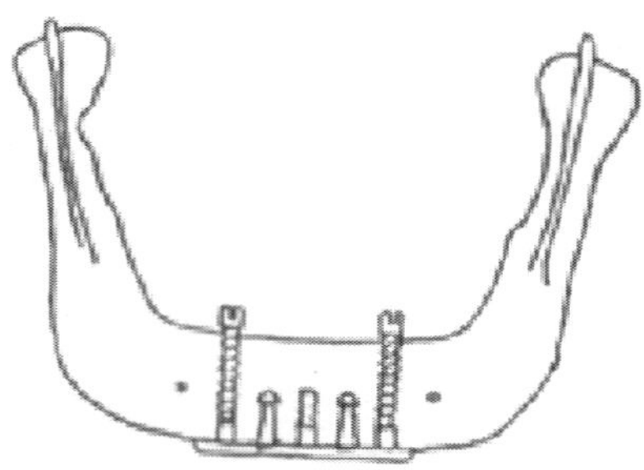

Figure 5. Transosseous Implants.

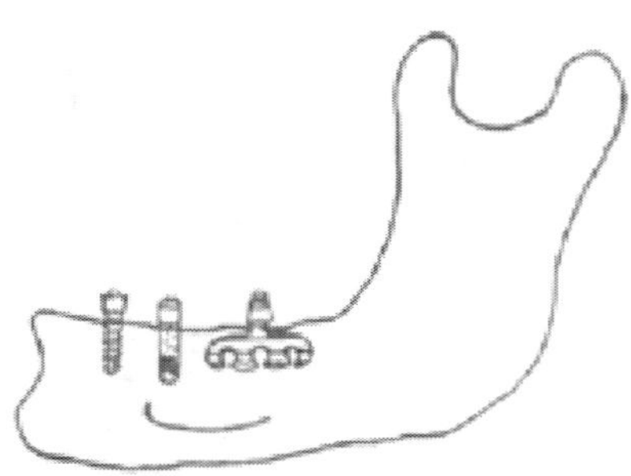

Figure 6. Endosseous Implants.

3. Endosseous Implants: These are partially submerged and anchored within the bone. These are the most commonly used. Various one-stage endosteal pins, screws and cylinder implant designs emerged in the early 1960's. The majority of these screw-shaped implants were one piece and were not submerged, they generally did not osseointegrate. Some workers theorized that the fibrous peri-implant membrane with it's shock absorbing feature was preferable to an implant fused to bone. We now know that this is not the case.

Configuration Design

According to the configuration design implants may be

- Root Form
- Blade Form

1. Root form implants:

These are screw type endosseous implants and has been derived due their cylindrical structure. A two-stage threaded titanium root-form implant was first presented in North America by *Branemark* in *1978* at a conference in Toronto [53]. Branemark [54] had found in conjunction with vital microscopy studies that titanium oculars placed in the femur of rabbits could not be removed from bone after a period of healing. Branemark developed and tested a two-stage dental implant system utilizing pure titanium screws, which he termed as *fixtures.*

The first fixtures were placed in patients in 1965, and intensive clinical studies have proceeded ever since. His well-documented, long-term prospective studies offered clear evidence of prolonged survival, freestanding function, bone maintenance and significant improvement in the benefit-to-risk ratio over all previous dental implants [55]. Osseointegration undoubtedly represents the most significant breakthrough in dentistry in the past 25 years. It has revolutionized dental treatment planning. With the Branemark implant came the concept of the premachined abutment and the fixed detachable prosthesis. Based on Branemark's extensive and weighty documentation of implant efficacy and safety and early replication by *Zarb* [56] and others, dental schools and dental specialities, which heretofore had avoided any involvement in this field, finally recongnized and incorporated dental implants into their curricula and training programs [57].

Subsequent to the Branemark implant, many other root-forms have been introduced and enjoy widespread clinical use [58]. Some are traditional screws (ITI-plasma sprayed); others have platinum forms rather than threads *(Stryker)* [59]; the IMZ implant is a press-fit stress broken titanium plasma-sprayed cylinder [60]; many are hollow cylinders *(ITI, Core-Vent)* [61-63]; and some are HA coated *(Integral, Calcitek, Inc.)* [64]. Plasma sprayed or other induced surface roughness enhances bone deposition and maintenance as well as affording an increased surface area for stress transfer [52].

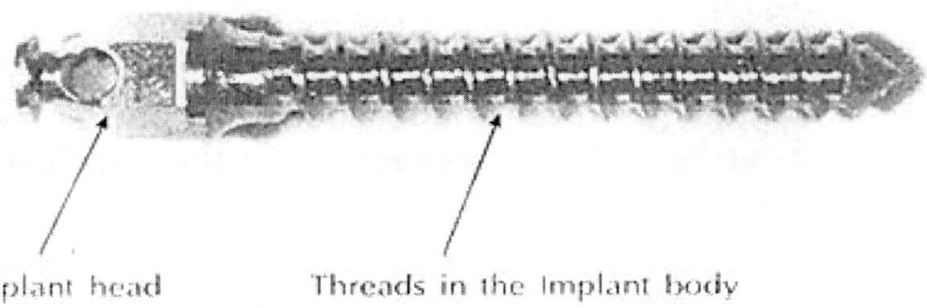

Figure 7. Root Form Implant.

2. Blade form implants:

In 1969, two variations of the blade implant were introduced independently by *Linkow* and *Roberts* [65]. Linkow subsequently designed a myriad of configurations for the blade, making it suitable for broad applicability in the maxilla and the mandible, especially for the placement in narrow ridges. It did require shared support with natural teeth and could not function on it's own. The blade implant was restorable within a month of placement and soon became the most widely used device in implantology.

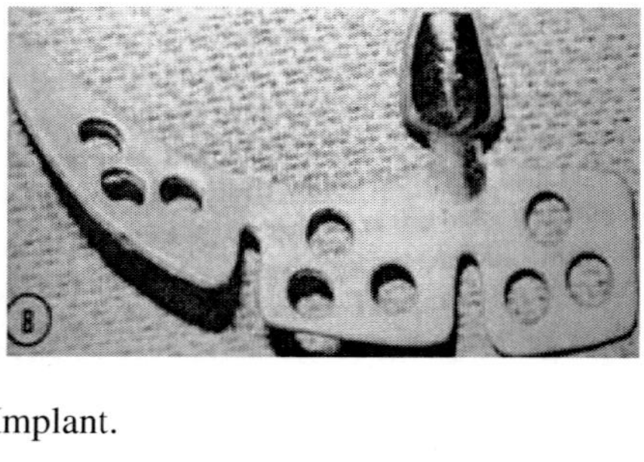

Figure 8. Blade Form Implant.

Implant Materials

According to the material the implant is made up of, it may be classified as:

(1) Stainless steel
(2) Cobalt chromium Molybdenum (Co-Cr-Mo)
(3) Titanium
(4) Ceramics.

Implant Surface Texture

Implants may be classified according to their surface texture as:

(1) Threaded
The root form implants are generally threaded as this provides for a greater surface area and stability of the implants.

(2) Non-threaded
The screw type implants are usually non porous, where as the plate or blade implants have vents in the implant body to aid in the bone growth and thus better interlocking between the metal structure and the surrounding bone.

Mode of Placement

Implants may be:

Self Tapping with Pre-drilling

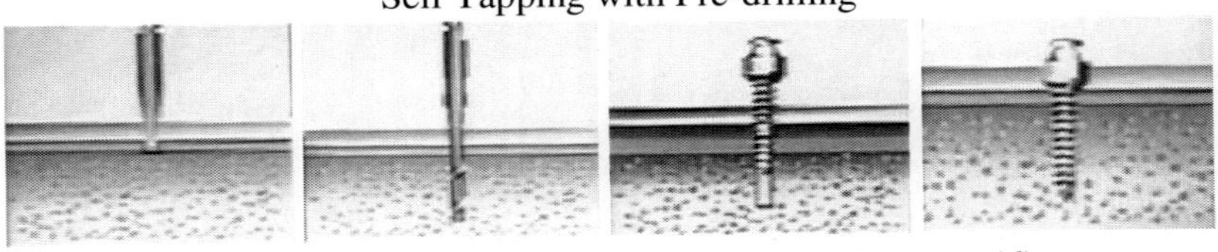

(a) (b) (c) (d)

Figure 9. Self Tapping with Pre-drilling Implant (a) Making of punch hole with the round bur (b) Drilling (c) Insertion of self tapping Implant (d) Complete Implant inserted into the bone.

In these type of implants, first a pilot hole is drilled using a bur and then the implant is screwed.

Self Drilling

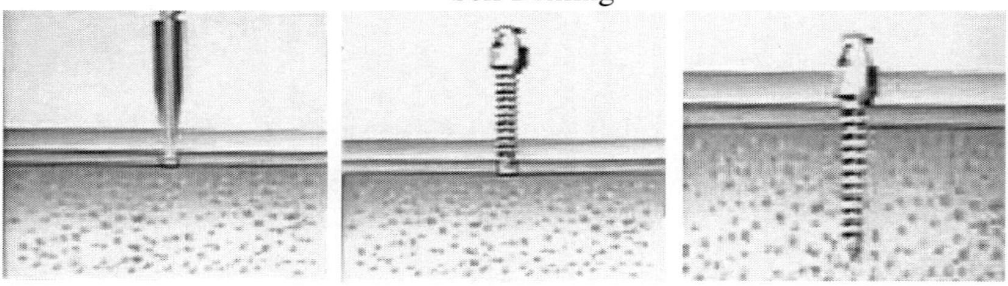

(a) (b) ©

Figure 10. Self Drilling Implant (a) Making of punch hole with the round bur (b) Introduction of self drilling Implant to the punch hole (c) Complete Implant inserted into the bone.

In these types of implants, the implant has a sharp head and it can be directly screwed in the bone without pre-drilling.

Chapter 5

Materials Used for Implants

In the 16th and 17th centuries gold and ivory dental implants were used [9].

Metal implant devices of gold, iridium, lead, tantalum; stainless steel and cobalt alloy were developed in the 20th century [66].

Cobalt-chromium-molybdenum sub periosteal and titanium blade implants were introduced in 1940 and 1950's. Nonmetal biomaterials [67-68] such as vitreous [69-70] and pyrolytic carbon, aluminium oxide, and hydroxyapatite were introduced in 1970's. In 1982 in Toronto, Branemark presented a work which he began 15 years back and the principles of osseointegration was set forth [71]. With osseointegration a clinical reality the root form implant once again became implantology most dominant design. A multitude of solid and hollow screw, and press fit forms developed with or without a titanium plasma forms developed with or without a titanium plasma spray or HA coating [72, 73, 74, 75]. The dentist's introduction to dental implants invariably includes an introduction to titanium. A successful long term implant requires biocompatibility, toughness, strength, corrosion resistance, wear resistance and fracture resistance.

Titanium

Titanium alloys of interest to dentistry exist in three forms:

1. Alpha
2. Beta
3. Alpha-beta phase (most commonly used)

The alloys most commonly used for dental implants are of the alpha-beta variety. Of these the most common ones contain 6% Aluminum and 4% vanadium (Ti-6Al-4V). After heat treatment these alloy possess many favorable physical and mechanical properties that make them excellent implant materials. They are light, strong and highly resistant to fatigue and corrosion. Although they are stiffer than bone, their modulus of elasticity (stiffness) is closer to bone than any other important implant metal (except pure Ti). This property leads to a more even distribution of stress at the critical bone-implant interface because the bone and implant will flex in a similar fashion and maintain the contact.

Ti and its alloys oxidize readily in air. This surface oxide is extremely stable in the physiologic environment of the body (ie) "passivity." If an implant metal is oxidized and the oxide does not breakdown under physiologic conditions the metal is said to be passive.

The stability and inertness of this surface oxide layer acts to protect Ti from corrosive breakdown when used in the body. The elimination of surface irregularities and contaminants is important when preparing a metal for implantation.

Titanium can be coupled with equally passive metals in the body without causing galvanic corrosion.

Chapter 6

Biocompatibility of Titanium Implants

1. Implant Preparation
2. Structure and Composition
3. Chemical Bonding and Chemical Processes at the Interface
4. Surface Roughness

Implant Preparation

In the procedure developed by Adell et al. [78] the implant is first prepared by, careful controlled mechanical shaping (lathing, threading and so forth) of the pure titanium raw material. During the machining procedure fresh metallic titanium is exposed to the atmosphere, consisting of air amid any added lubricant and/or coolant. The air exposure of the machined surface results in extremely rapid oxide formation. For example, in less than a millisecond an oxide layer greater than 10 A^{o} is formed, and within a minute the oxide thickness will be of the order of 50 to 100 A^{o}. The actual thickness, composition, and microstructure of the oxide will depend on several factors, including the pressure and speed of machining, which in turn determine the surface temperature. Considerable variations in surface (oxide) properties may therefore be expected with different machining conditions.

The next preparation steps consists of ultrasonic cleaning and autoclaving. The latter procedure involves additional growth of the surface oxide, as well as, probable incorporation of OH radicals in the oxide. The prepared implant is then ready for it's surgical installation.

Structure and Composition

The important fact that the implant surface consists of a relatively thick titanium oxide must be remembered when the chemistry at the implant-tissue interface is considered. The chemical properties, and therefore the interface chemistry, are determined by the oxide layer and not by the metal itself. This is a general statement that applies to all metallic implant materials (with a possible exception of gold and platinum) and is significant since there is no similarity whatsoever among the physical, chemical, and mechanical properties of a metal and it's oxide. Some metallic implants, and particularly titanium, could actually be viewed as composite materials where the advantageous mechanical properties of the metal are combined with the desirable surface chemical properties of the oxide. From a biochemical viewpoint titanium implants could therefore be regarded as oxide ceramics.

The bulk of the titanium metal is covered by a dense oxide film with a thickness of approximately 100 A^o. Because surface oxides grow by inward transport of oxygen atoms (from O_2 molecules or H_2O in the atmosphere) and/or outward metal atom transport from the metal-oxide interface, there will be some concentration gradients for oxygen and titanium. An oxide formed in this way will be quite different from the corresponding bulk oxide, with expectations for a high degree of nonstoichiometry, variations in crystal structure, and richness of defects in the surface oxide, which will have consequences for the interface chemistry. Titanium forms several stable oxides such as TiO_2, TiO and TiO_3, with TiO_2 being the most common one. All oxides have high dielectric constants (higher than for most other metal oxides) in the range of 50 to 120. For these reasons single stoichiometric oxide is not expected to form on the implant surface. Lacking a better chemical characterization, the oxide might be called TiO_x, where x gives the average oxygen content of the oxide.

Chemical Bonding and Chemical Processes at the Interface

Chemical Bonding

The first monomolecular layer of biomolecules that bond to the oxide of the implant surface has not yet been identified. There are several types of bonding by which the biomolecules may stick to the implant surface. These include the long-range but weak Van-der Waal interaction and the short-range strong chemical bonding (e.g., ionic and covalent bonding). In the former case the bond strengths are of the order of 1-10 Kcal/mol, which are *so small that permanent bonds are not established* at body temperature. If this type of bonding is dominant, there is continuous and rapid exchange of the biomolecules that stick to the surface. The presence of water molecules is, of course, important both in modifying the bond strengths and in establishing the bonds. For Vander Waal's bonding, the dielectric constant of the implant surface and the polarizability of the molecule or radical group that binds to the surface are important physical parameters that determine the bond strength.The high dielectric constant of the titanium oxides may thus be a crucial factor that distinguishes titanium from other metal implants.

The second class of bonding is due to the overlapping charge clouds of the surface and the adsorbing molecules. It is characterized by it's short range (approximate atomic dimensions), often a high degree of directionality (as in covalent bonds) and the possibility of high bond strengths. Typical values are in the range of 10-100 Kcal/mol. For bond strengths greater than 30 Kcal/mol the bonding can be regarded as irreversible since the half-life for molecule exchange will then be several years. For this type of bonding, the local (on the angstrom scale) composition of the surface is important. The variations in local microstructure along the oxide surface represent a spectrum of bond strengths and geometries to which different biomolecules will have widely different affinities.

In summary, an oxidized metal implant surface offers a wide range of bond strengths and chemical bonding types. In view of the large spectrum of biomolecules exposed to the surface, it is likely that several of these bonding situations are established: *some representing irreversible bonding and some characterized by continuous exchange of molecules, that is, a dynamic equilibrium.*

Chemical Processes

An investigation of the thickness of the surface oxide as a function of the implant period indicates that the oxide thickness increases much faster at the implant position in bone than when it is left in air. This growth must take place by either or both of the two mechanisms namely, metal atom/ion diffusion out to the oxide surface followed by oxidation, or oxygen diffusion from an oxygen-carrying species at the oxide surface to the metal oxide interface. As a result of participation of hydrogen atoms (or protons), the oxide can also grow by hydroxide formation. Other components that can contribute to growth and modification of the oxide include the mineral ions of Ca and P.

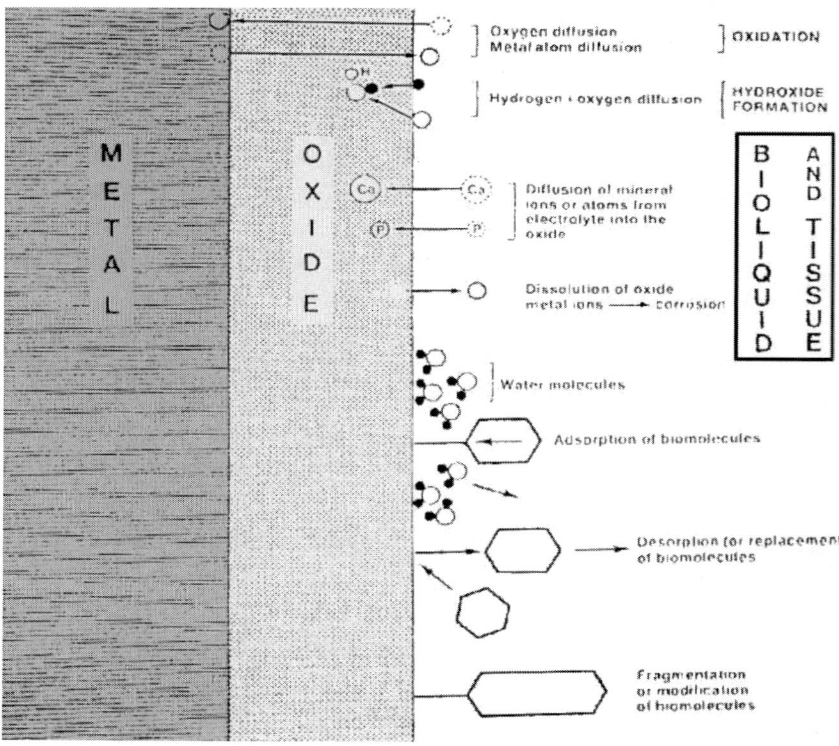

Figure 11. Chemical processes at the Titanium Implant – Tissue Interface.

The possibility of dissolution of the protecting oxide layer (corrosion), may be a severe problem with some implant materials. This appears to be a very slow process with titanium, probably due to the high stability of it's oxide. However, quantitative measurements of the "corrosion" rate are needed. Hydration of the oxide is another process that is likely to occur and that maybe important in establishing a suitable chemical environment for the biomolecules.

For some combinations of local surface composition and biomolecule, the chemical interaction may be so strong that a chemical bond is broken *within* the molecule. Even if the bond is incompletely broken, it may be modified to the extent that the molecule itself undergoes a considerable change in it's biochemical properties. Changes such as denaturing of proteins may of course be harmful for the future development of the interface zone. Recent experiments on titanium implants suggest the possibility that organic material is incorporated in the surface oxide under in vivo conditions.

Surface Roughness

It is suitable to divide the discussion into two parts: one dealing with surface roughness where the surface curvature is always much larger than atomic dimensions and one where the surface is rough on an atomic scale. In the former part the main role of surface roughness is that it can improve the mechanical strength of an implant situation, for example, by a more advantageous stress distribution. The chemical bonding etc., will be unaffected by roughness on this scale (approximately equal to or greater than 1 micrometer).

A surface roughness on the atomic scale can, on the contrary, also influence the (local) chemical bonding through the particular geometric arrangements that can be established. When van der waals interaction is prevailing, surface roughness will be in principle also modify the interaction since it influences the local electromagnetic fields at the surface.

Surface-Active Ceramics

Glass ceramics, such as Bioglass and Cervital, are polycrystalline ceramics produced by the controlled crystallization of glasses. Table 1 shows the chemical composition of glass ceramic materials.

Table 1. Chemical composition of Glass Ceramic Materials

Compound	Mole %		Weight
	Bioglass 42S5.6	Bioglass 45S5	Cervital Bioactive
SiO_2	42.1	46.1	40.0-50.0
CaO	29.0	26.9	30.0-35.0
NaO_2	26.3	24.4	5.0-10.0
P_2O_3	2.6	2.6	10.0-15.0
MgO	-	-	2.5-5.0
K_2O	-	-	0.5-3.0

Glass ceramics have poor mechanical properties for load carrying applications because they are extremely brittle. Controlling grain size, however, increases both tensile strength by a factor of two (from 100 to 200 MPa) and abrasion resistance. The implant surface responds to local pH changes by releasing sodium ions in exchange for phosphorus or hydrogen ions. A calcium phosphate layer forms on the surface. Osteoblasts proliferate at the surface, and collagen fibrils become incorporated into the calcium phosphate - rich layer.

Calcium phosphate ceramics, classified as polycrystalline ceramics, have a material structure derived from individual crystals that have become fused at the grain boundaries during high-temperature sintering processes. Hydroxyapatite (HA), $(Ca_{10}(PO_4)_6(OH)_2]$, commonly called tribasic calcium phosphate, is a geologic mineral in vertebrate bone tissue. Tribasic calcium phosphate should not be confused with other calcium phosphate ceramics, especially tricalcium phosphate (TCP), $[Ca_3(PO_4)_2]$ which is chemically similar to HA but is not a natural bone mineral.

The biocompatibility of the calcium phosphate ceramics is well documented. The body's typical response to these implanted ceramics is:

1. No local or systemic toxicity.
2. No inflammatory or foreign body reaction.
3. Functional integration with bone.
4. No alteration to natural mineralization processes.
5. Chemical bonding to bone via natural bone cementing mechanisms.

The biocompatibility and close chemical composition to natural bone mineral are factors that make the calcium phosphate ceramics desirable bioactive materials. HA implant surfaces have been characterized as being capable of forming direct, intimate bonds with the surrounding bone. The bonding area (approximately 500 to 200 Å) contains biologic apatite crystals that are highly oriented at the interface with a 100 Å periodicity similar to that of calcified tissue, as determined by electron diffraction studies. The bone apatite crystals are arranged against the implant surface in a palisade fashion, resembling the natural bonding between two bone fragments. The bonding area contains a ground substance that is heavily mineralized, although devoid of collagen fibrils, and has been likened to the natural bone-cementing substance. The natural bone-cementing substance is amorphous in structure, heavily mineralized, and rich in mucopolysaccharides. Because the bond area contains a substance biologically similar to the natural bone cement substance, it is reasonable that the bond between bone and the calcium phosphate ceramic is strong.

Chapter 7

Implant Design Properties

A common method of implant fixation is impaction into the alveolar ridge. The implants are held in place by compressive stress interaction, and the devices are designed to remain in compression relative to the surrounding tissue. Static and dynamic masticatory forces are then transmitted from the implant to the surrounding tissues. The precision required to obtain uniform contact between the device and surrounding bone is limited by the skills of the surgeon and design of the instrumentation with which the site is prepared. The surface area of actual contact is probably small relative to the implant surface area. These contact points tend to induce areas of stress concentrations rather than an even distribution of stresses. Bone maintains its structural integrity by responding to stress; high areas of stress concentration are often associated with bone resorption. Additionally, fibrous encapsulations of varying thicknesses are common occurrences that further alter the ability of the implant to distribute stress uniformly. This situation often manifests itself in eventual implant loosening and migration, leading to patient discomfort and the need for eventual removal.

Several types of implant fixation methods and surface texture designs have been investigated to obtain better surgical fit and stress distribution at the implant-bone interface. These methods include direct bone apposition to the implant surface, bone growth into porous-surfaced implants, and chemical bonding between bone and surface-active chemical implant coatings.

Direct Bone Apposition

Optimal osseointegration at the bone-implant interface is affected by the material properties and design of the implant. Implant design encompasses both the surface texture and geometry of the implant. The mechanical properties of the implant-bone interface have been investigated with various surface preparations: smooth finish, roughened or grit-blasted finishes and grooved surfaces. Histologically, implants with smooth finishes have interfaces characterized by fibrous encapsulation, whereas implants with grit-blasted finishes have interfaces characterized by areas of direct bone apposition. Several studies determined that surface texture is a significant factor in obtaining adequate implant fixation with direct bone apposition methods.

The effects of implant diameter and length on direct bone apposition have been studied using a dental implant model.

Mechanical results indicate a statistical correlation with implant length and no correlation with implant diameter. Implications of factors involving cortical and cancellous bone structural differences are attributed to some of the mechanical differences between implant lengths.

Porous Ingrowth Attachment

It is generally accepted that an implant can achieve stabilization by tissue growth into the surface porous structure if the material is bioinert, if there is direct apposition of the bone at the implant interface, if there is a minimal or no movement at the implant site, and if the porous structure has appropriate pore size and morphology. The effectiveness of porous coatings as a means of biologic fixation becomes apparent when considering interfacial mechanical properties. The interface attachment strength of porous implants relying on bone ingrowth for fixation are at least an order of magnitude higher than that of nonporous implants relying on direct bone apposition for fixation. Several different porous structures have been evaluated: irregular, fiber mesh and bead; however, bead porous coatings have been studied in more detail than the other types.

Calcium Phosphate Ceramic Coatings

HA-coated and uncoated dental implants have been evaluated in dog models to compare both mechanical and histologic response. The grit-blasted implants demonstrated osseointegration after 4 months' implantation. Even at 10 months, however, the bone was not continuous at the implant interface. The HA-coated implants exhibited direct bonding of bone to the HA surface at 1 month. By 4 months, lamellar bone was observed at the HA-bone interface.

HA-coated and grit-blasted titanium dental implants were evaluated 6 weeks after implantation into healed extraction sites. Implants were mechanically tested to determine interface torsional strength. Mechanical results demonstrated an interface torsional strength of 3.98 ± 0.93 MPa for HA-coated implants and 2.25 ± 0.65 MPa for grit-blasted implants. The difference in torsional strengths was statistically significant. Histologically, HA-coated implants exhibited direct bone apposition with no intervening fibrous tissue at the implant interface. Although the grit-blasted implants also exhibited regions of direct bone apposition, these regions were limited to a small percentage of the implant surface.

Optimizing Biologic Attachment Methods

Optimal attachment at the bone-implant interface is affected by the material properties and design of the implant. Other conditions that affect osseointegration are instrumentation design, surgical technique, initial implant stability, and direct contact with the surrounding bone.

Motion at Bone-Implant Interface

Persistent micromotion at the bone-implant interface has been an established cause of bone resorption and necrosis. Necrosis and destructive bone remodeling often result in fibrous tissue infiltration at the interface and may cause implant loosening. Also, any initial gap between the implant and surrounding bone may adversely alter the amount and rate at which osseointegration occurs. Initial implant stability is essential for early tissue infiltrate within the porous structure to differentiate into bone by either direct bone formation or appositional bone growth. When excessive early movement occurs at the bone-implant interface, bone formation within the pores is inhibited. The majority of research concerning motion at the interface has involved porous implants; however, the findings are applicable for press-fit implant systems.

It is generally accepted that micromotion of 150 um is the upper limit of acceptable motion. In a carefully controlled study, Bragdon et al. (1991) determined that 150 um of implant motion did not allow bone ingrowth.

Surgical Fit

The technical difficulties is cutting bone precisely to provide an exact fit around the implant often result in a poor surgical fit. Difficulties in achieving initial implant-bone interface apposition are due to implant and instrumentation design and surgical technique. Numerous researchers have investigated the effect of interface gap spaces on the histologic response to implants. These studies demonstrate that the closer the fit between the bone and the implant (< 0.5 mm) the earlier osseointegration is achieved and the quality of bone is superior.

Surgical fit is also a concern for HA-coated prostheses because HA coatings do not make up for improper surgical placement of the implant. The concentrations of the physiologic components necessary for bone formation are decreased across large interfacial gaps as compared with concentrations for press-fit situations. Therefore the rate of gap filling, and subsequent ingrowth, is delayed. Large gaps may reduce the quality of bone at the interface as compared with that of press-fit interfaces.

In summary, the mechanical and chemical properties of metals, such as titanium and titanium-based alloys and cobalt-based alloys, and ceramics, such as glass and calcium phosphate, make them suitable for implant applications. Several factors, however, affect the biologic response to these implanted materials. The predominant tissue found at the implant interface is affected by implant stability, material biocompatibility and implant design and placement into the surgical site. Improvements in implant design and surface preparation may increase.

Chapter 8

Factors Influencing Osseointegration

Important factors to ensure a reliable bone anchorage of an implanted device

1. Implant biocompatibility
2. Design characteristics
3. Surface characteristics
4. State of the host bed
5. Surgical technique
6. Loading conditions.

Implant Biocompatibility

Commercially pure titanium, niobium and possibly tantalum are known to be most well accepted in bone tissue because of their adherent self repairing oxide layer which has excellent resistance to corrosion.

Hydroxyapatite coated implants has a greatest advantage because this material elicits a more rapid bone response than uncoated metals (particularly in case of poor bone beds).

But the risk associated with it is gradual coat loss – bone saucerisation-implant instability. Others like copper, silver have poor biocompatibility.

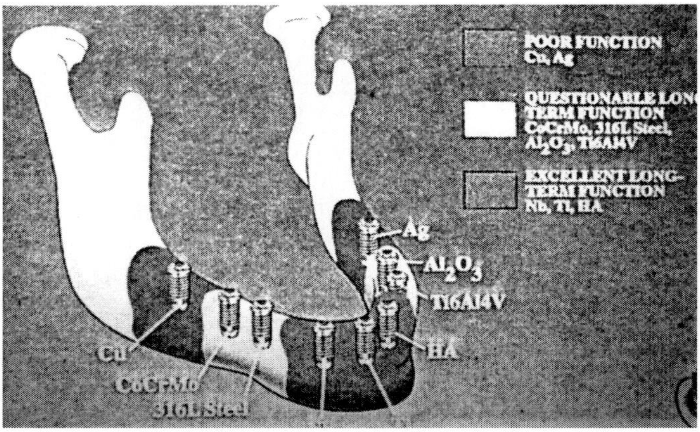

Figure 12. Biocompatibility of the Mandibular bone with different Implant materials.

Implant Design

Threaded type of implants have good stability than non threaded and cylindrical type.

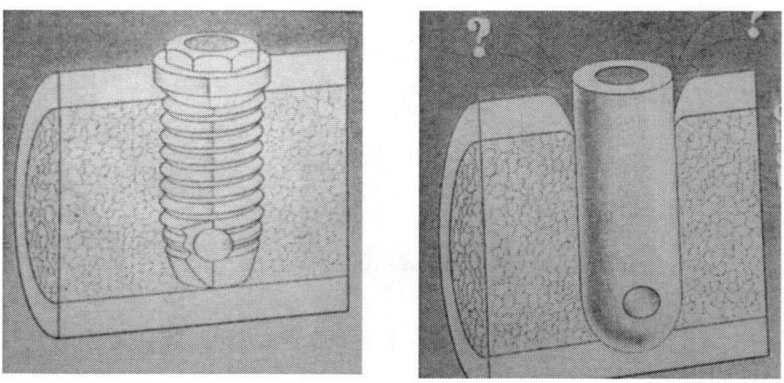

(a) (b)

Figure 13. Implant Designs (a) Threaded Implant (b) Non- threaded Implant.

Implant Surface

Implants with smooth surface do not result in an acceptable bone cell adhesion. Some microirregularities are necessary for proper cell adhesion.

High ionic reactions and chemical bonds increase surface energy improving the cellular attachment thereby increasing the implant stability.

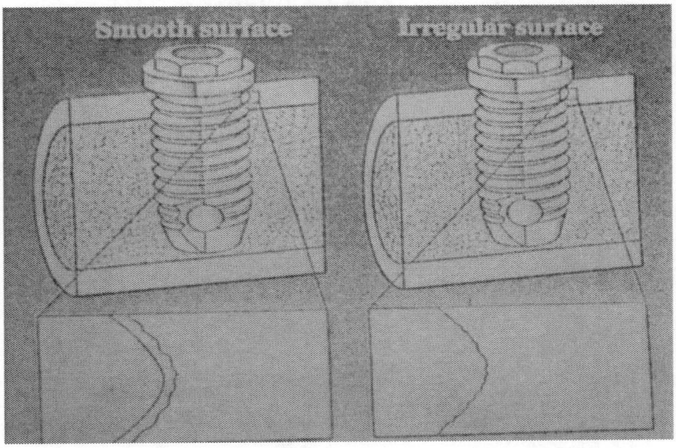

(a) (b)

Figure 14. Implant Surface (a) Smooth surface Implant (b) Irregular surface Implant.

State of the Host Bed

Ideal host bed should be healthy and with adequate bone stocks. Bone exposed to irradiation, ridge height resorption and osteoporosis are undesirable states for implantation prognosis.

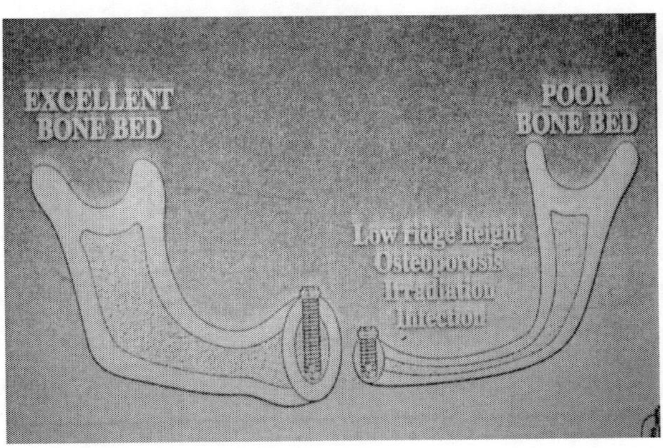

Figure 15. Types of bone bed.

Surgical Technique

The critical time/temperature relationship for bone tissue necrosis is around 47°C applied for 1 min more or less simultaneously to achieve the desirable goal of a direct bone anchorage.

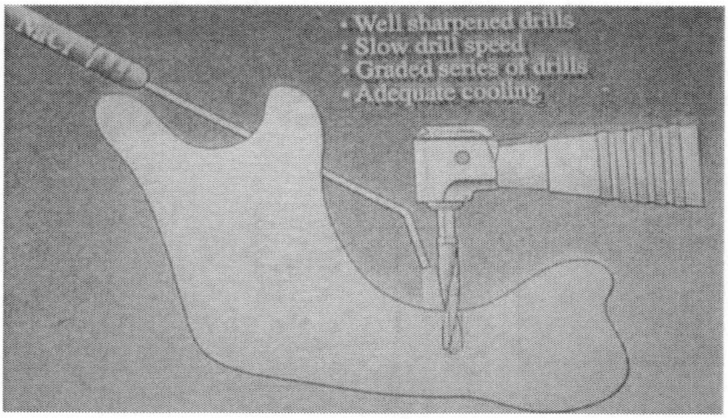

Figure 16. Ideal surgical technique.

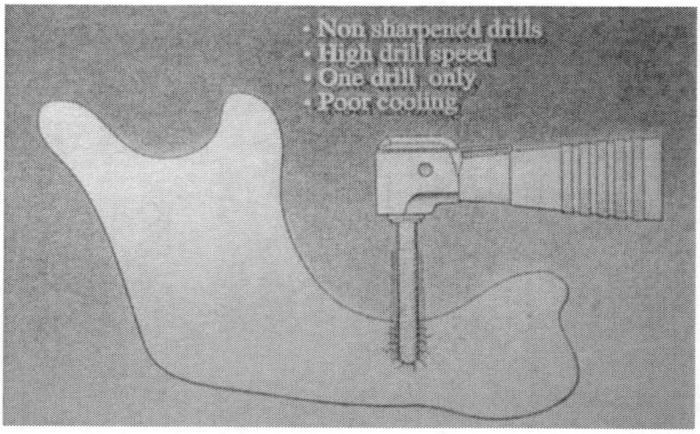

Figure 17. Poor surgical technique.

Loading Conditions

Implant in early remodeling phase will be surrounded by soft tissue. Initially after implant insertion it will be sensitive to loading – increased soft tissue formation – permanent soft tissue anchorage similar to fracture. Length of time loading should be avoided is dependant on the implantation site as well as on the bone bed quality. Branemark with his controlled implant system advocated use of 3 month loading delay in the mandible and 4-6 months delay in maxilla.

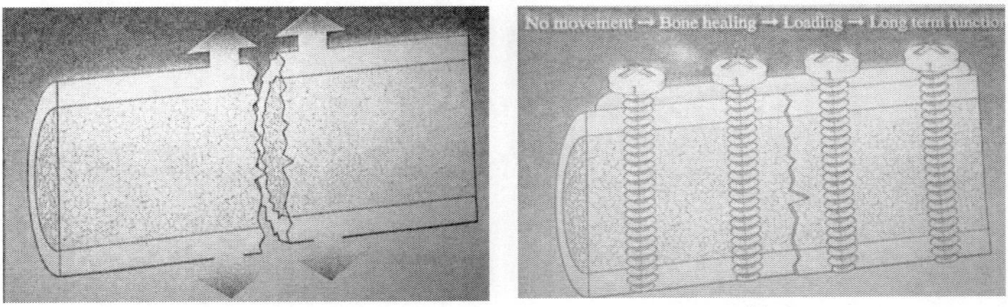

(a) (b)

Figure 18. Loading Conditions (a) Non- ideal moving area (b) Ideal loading immovable area.

Chapter 9

Healing of Endosseous Implants

During the past two decades, endosseous implants have been used extensively to achieve osseointegration for prosthetic rehabilitation of edentulism.

Generally a surgical procedure is performed on a patient to insert a foreign material into bone, and then the body is called on the "heal" the wound. Since the mid - 1970s, the general consensus for successful implant healing shifted toward that of a direct bond of the implant to bone with no intervening fibrous tissue, i.e., osseous integration.

There are many requirements for successful osseous integration that must be considered during the placement of endosseous implants. This section discusses the general healing of bone and soft tissues around implants, factors influencing healing, biocompatibility of materials, and the healing response of hard and soft tissue with implants.

Bone Healing

After the surgical placement of implants into enosteal locations, the traumatized bone around these implants begins the process of wound healing, which can be separated into the inflammatory phase, the proliferative phase, and the maturation phase (Table 2).

Table 2. Phases of Generalized Bone Healing

Phase	Timing	Specific Occurrence
1. Inflammatory phase	Day 1-10	Adsorption of plasma proteins Platelet aggregation and activation Clotting cascade activation Cytokine release Nonspecific cellular inflammatory response Specific cellular inflammatory response Macrophage-mediated inflammation
2. Proliferative phase	Day 3-27	Neovascularization Differentiation, proliferation, and activation of cells Production of immature connective tissue matrix
3. Maturation phase	After day 28	Remodeling of the immature bone matrix with coupled resorption/deposition of bone Bone remodeling in response to implant loading Physiologic bone resorption.

Bone-Implant Interface

The type of interface that develops between the implant and bone depends on many variables. Ultrastructural investigations between implants and bone in areas of osseous integration reveal a zone of amorphous material between the implant and bone. The exact chemical nature of interface that forms between the amorphous layer and the metallic implant surface is yet to be determined. It has been theorized, however, that weak Van der Waals bonding, direct chemical bonding (i.e., ionic, covalent), or a combination of the two many be present. The implant material in question is the most important factor that determines the chemical nature of this interface. Chemical bonding of the implant material to the surrounding bone is a well-described phenomenon with certain materials, such as calcium phosphate ceramics. Other materials, such as alloys, carbon, aluminum oxide, and most polymers, have a minimal to nonexistent interfacial chemical bonding, but they have excellent bone contact. It is controversial, however, whether commercially pure titanium forms a direct chemical bond to bone but it is believed that although a chemical bond may be persent, the bond strength is of a lesser magnitude than that experienced with HA. Table 3 summarizes some of the commonly used implant materials and their bond type to bone. Table 4 describes the degree of compatibility and tissue reaction to specific material.

Table 3. Biomaterial summary of surface and interface properties

Biomaterial	Surface	Active (A) or Passive (P)	Bonded (B) or Not (N) to Bone
Metals			
Re-Cr-Ni	Cr_xO_y	P	N
Ti and Ti-6A-4v	TiO2	A-P	B
Co alloys	Cr_xO_y	P	N
Ceramics and Carbons			
Al_2O_3	Al_2O_3	P	N
HA	$Ca_{10}(PO_4)_6(OH)_2$	A	B
TCP and ALCAP	$CaPO_4$	A	B
Bioglass or Ceravital	$CaPO_4$	A	B
C and C-Si	C or C-Si	P	N
Polymers & Composites			
Polyethylene	Polymer	P	N
Dacron	Polymer	P	N
Polytetrafluoroethylene	Polymer	P	N
Polymethylmethacrylate	Polymer	P	N
Silicone rubber	Polymer	P	N
Polysulfone	Polymer	P	N
Composites	Polymer	P	N

Table 4. Grouping of Hard Tissue Replacement Materials According to Their Compatibility to Bony Tissue

Degree of compatibility	Characteristics of Reaction of Bony Tissue	Materials
Biotolerant	Implants separated from adjacent bone by a soft tissue layer along most of the interface: distance osteogenesis	Stainless steel; PMMA bone cements; CoCrMo and CoCr MoNi alloys
Bioinert	Direct contact to bony tissue: contact osteogenesis	Alumina ceramics, zirconia ceramics, titanium, tantalum, niobium, carbon
Bioactive	Bonding to bony tissue: bonding osteogenisis	Calcium phosphate-containing glasses, glass ceramics, ceramics, titanium

Mucoperiosteal-Implant Interface

Dental implants have the unique feature of penetrating through lining epithelium. Establishment of an adequate connective tissue seal around an implant provides a barrier to the ingress of oral toxins and bacteria into the internal environment. Some authors believe that maintenance of this seal is essential for preventing the initial peri-implant tissue inflammation that can lead to eventual destruction of implant support. Ten Cate [80] indicates that lack of a biologic seal will not doom implants to failure, but rather the connective tissue response is more likely to be the critical factor involved in implant loss.

Epithelial regeneration around well-integrated implants results in a structure similar to the gingival tissues around natural teeth. The keratinized oral epithelium is continuous with nonkeratinized sulcular epithelium adjacent to the implant in the peri-implant sulcus. This sulcus is analogous to the periodontal sulcus around natural teeth and is approximately 3 to 4 mm deep in healthy sites. Junctional epithelium is located in the portion of the sulcus, and this portion of the epithelium is adherent to the implant surface. Ultrastructural investigations of this attachment reveal that the junctional epithelial cells attach to the implant surface with a basal lamina and hemidesmosomes in the same way that they would attach to teeth. The basal lamina-hemidesmosomal complex is thought to be chemically bonded to the implant surface by a 10- to 20-nm amorphous glycoprotein layer similar to that found at the bone-implant interface. These hemidesmosomes become evident 2 to 3 days after implant insertion.

Factors Affecting Healing

There are many factors that can affect the healing process. Some of these factors deal with surgical technique and treatment protocol, whereas others deal with patient selection, hygiene, loading pattern, and site selection.

Surgical Technique

All surgical procedures are considered to be traumatic to the host tissues, but the level of trauma induced is one of the critical factors that determines whether healing will progress toward fibrous or osseous integration. Studies by Albrektsson [81] reveal that all surgical preparations on hard tissue cause a necrotic zone of bone at the implant bone interface owing to cutting of blood vessels, frictional heat generated during instrumentation, and vibrational trauma. Excessive trauma, however, invariably leads to fibrous encapsulation of the implant. Surgical trauma must be minimized during all aspects of implant surgery to optimize success rates.

Surgical instrumentation of bone produces heat that can elevate the local temperature of bone. Rotary instruments used during preparation of an implant site can cause bone necrosis that can impair local bone viability and eventually lead to fibrous encapsulation of the implant. In vivo studies have shown that traumatic surgical manipulation of bone causes poor vascularization of the implant border zone with delay or absence of ossification. The effect of elevated temperature of bone tissue has been postulated to cause denaturation of alkaline phosphatase, which occurs at 56°C. The crucial threshold temperature for impaired bone regeneration, however, has been shown to be as low as 44°C to 47°C when applied to the bone for periods of 1 minute. Possible explanations for this lower critical temperature threshold could possibly be interference with local circulation, capillary leakage, and dehydration and osmotic changes that occur with traumatic manipulation of bone. These effects could cause enough of a change in bone physiology to result in altered differentiation of local progenitor cells, leading to fibrous encapsulation.

Bone temperatures of 60ºC can be found during bone surgery using conventional instrumentation even with copious external irrigation. It has been shown, however, that gentle surgical technique using a graduated series of sharp drills run intermittently at low speeds with copious amounts of internal and external irrigation can help to maintain the local bone temperature below the crucial threshold. This allows for the escape of debris from the bur flutes during preparation, which minimizes frictional heat and enables and irrigant to control local temperatures effectively. It is probably most critical that ultraslow rotary instrumentation (15 to 30 rpm) be used for the final phase of implant site preparation (tapping).

Delicate manipulation of soft tissue around the implant site must also be observed during implant placement. Maintenance of periosteal integrity allows for preservation of local osteoblastic function and maximization of local bone vascularity, which is essential for implant healing to occur.

Premature Loading

As mentioned previously, surgical preparation of bone for the placement of implants inevitably causes a zone of necrotic bone around the implant as a result of the surgical procedure. This zone of dead bone must be resorbed and replaced by new vascularized bone for osseous integration to occur. Significant movement of implants during this healing phase has been shown to result in fibrous encapsulation by inhibiting new bone formation and by inhibiting revascularization of necrotic bone. Implant motion has been shown to activate local macrophages, causing them to release cytokines, eicosanoids, and metalloproteinases. It can also create conditions that promote wear and corrosion of the implant material, yielding particulate debris and metal ions. This can further activate inflammatory cells to elaborate other cytokines and enzymes, with the net effect being altered differentiation of local mesenchymal cells, leading to bone resorption and fibrous encapsulation.

Bone remodeling that occurs during the healing phase occurs at different rates, depending on the amount of local bone necrosis, local bone physiology, and generalized physical composition of the patient. For this reason, it is recommended that these implants remain in an unloaded state for a period of 2 to 8 months, depending on the clinical situation, implant material used, location of implantation, and whether the implant is placed into bone grafts.

Surgical Fit

Technical difficulties and inconsistencies between an implant and instrument diameter make it virtually impossible to obtain perfect microscopic contact between bone and implants. Even in the best situation, bone contacts only portions of the implant. When implants are placed into fresh extraction sockets, inconsistencies between the implant diameter and the tooth root diameter at the crest of the alveolar ridge create the potential for a significant space between the residual bone and the implant surface. Successful integration of the implant requires that bone be deposited in these areas for implant support.

Carlsson et al. (1988) [82] studied bone regeneration around titanium implants with interfacial gaps of 0, 0.35, and 0.85 mm. They demonstrated that even after 6 weeks the only implants to achieve significant osseous integration were the ones without interfacial gaps. In an animal investigation examining the healing of a 1-mm interfacial gap with HA-coated implants and titanium implants. Soballe et al. (1990) [83] demonstrated that there was significantly more bone contact with HA-coated implants than with titanium implants at a 4-week interval. These results would seem to indicate that longer healing periods may be required before loading implants when surgical fit is less than optimal and that earlier loading may be possible when using HA-coated implants.

Bone Quality

Bone quality and quantity are factors that can affect implant integration. There are significant differences between bone of the mandible and that of the maxilla. Within each of these bones, different bone quality is seen in different locations. The mandible generally has a denser cortex and coarser, thicker cancelli than does the maxilla. Bone in more posterior locations of both jaws tends to have a thinner, more porous cortex and finer cancelli. If implants are placed in bone with a dense cortex and a thick cancellous component, initial stabilization is more likely to be obtained when compared with implants placed in areas of thinner cortex with fine cancelli. As already seen, stable implants are more likely to heal with osseous integration than implants that are mobile. In addition, regeneration of a cortical rim of bone around the implant from the surrounding cancellous bone is more likely to progress at a faster rate if the surrounding bone is more dense. Thus, before functional loading, it is recommended that the implant healing period be anywhere from 2 to 8 months, depending on the quality of bone at the surgical site, implant material used, and whether the implant is placed into bone grafts. Differences in bone architecture are one of the reasons for the differences in success rates experienced between mandibular and maxillary implants.

Physical Condition of the Patient

The healing of implants involves a dynamic process in which the physical condition of a patient may alter the course of events. There are certain local and systemic conditions that have been implicated in causing impaired implant healing which have been listed below:

- Nutritional Status
- Aging
- Diabetes Mellitus
- Hematologic Derangements
- Corticosteroids
- Radiation

Chapter 10

Restorative Considerations in Combined Orthodontic Implant Therapy

Principles of Esthetics

The element of implant treatment in which the orthodontist can influence the restorative result is esthetics, particularly in the gingival area around the implants. To understand the orthodontist's role in the final gingival esthetic result, it is necessary to understand what effects the facial and inter-proximal tissue heights have on implants and teeth.

It is clear that the overlying gingival form reflects the underlying bone fairly accurately. Evaluating the differences between bony levels surrounding implants and those surrounding teeth provides a starting point for understanding the gingival differences. On natural teeth, there is a highly scalloped nature to alveolar bone from facial to interproximal to facial. This bony scallop essentially follow the rise and fall of the cementoenamel junction (CEJ), creating a dip of approximately 3 mm from facial to interproximal in the anterior teeth and decreasing as the CEJ flattens out on the posterior teeth. In contrast, an implant has no bony scallop from facial to interproximal since the heads of the implant systems are flat rather than scalloped like CEJ. Because of this, even if the bone were appropriately scalloped, placing the head of an implant flush with the interproximal bone would leave threads exposed on the facial surface of the implant that would not be covered by bone.

Conversely, if the implant were seated completely so that the facial bone covered the head of the implant, it would leave unsupported bone coronal to the head of the implant interproximally. This unsupported bone would resorb, removing the underlying support for what would have been the papilla. Because of these bony differences, it is extremely difficult to obtain a normal gingival scallop around multiple implants when compared with natural teeth. This difference is amplified by the differences in gingival height from facial to interproximal on natural teeth as compared with implants.

On natural teeth, a "biologic band" of connective tissue and epithelial attachment occupies an area on average 2 mm in height above the bone facially and interproximally. Coronal to the attachment, the average sulcus depth of the facial surface is 1 mm, leaving 3 mm of total gingival height above bone on the facial surfaces. Interproximally, however, there is an average sulcus depth of 2.5mm coronal to the attachment, resulting in a papilla height of 4.5 mm above bone. This 1.5 mm difference in gingival height above bone from facial to interproximal, when combined with the average 3-mm osseous scallop, results in an average gingival scallop of 4.5 mm from facial to interproximal. In other words, the tip of the papilla is located 4.5 mm more coronal than the facial free gingival margin. These numbers are of course averages that vary depending on the shape of the teeth and the nature of the periodontium, e.g., flat and thick versus scalloped and thin.

The challenge in managing the esthetics between implants in the anterior is twofold. First, bone between the implants is not as highly scalloped as it is around natural anterior teeth. This alone will result in a reduction in gingival scallop. In addition, the height differences (above bone) between facial and interproximal gingiva do not appear to be the same as that of natural teeth. As stated above, the average papilla on natural teeth is 4.5mm above the bone compared with 3 mm for the facial gingival. The actual tissue height around implants appears to range from 2mm to 4 mm depending on several factors, but with little difference between facial and interproximal. Therefore, for multiple implants side by side, the papilla is often only 1 mm to 2 mm more coronal than the facial free gingival margin, compared with 4.5 mm for natural teeth, so there can be almost no gingival scallop. This flat-looking gingival appearance is especially unaesthetic in the anterior region.

Of the team members, the orthodontist is the one who can take a two-tooth pontic site and convert it into two single-tooth implant sites via tooth movement e.g., a patient missing maxillary lateral incisors and first premolars.

A male patient [89] had congenitally missing multiple teeth, including the maxillary lateral incisors and premolars. The permanent canines had erupted next to the central incisors. One option would have been to leave the canines in the position and restore or reshape them to look like lateral incisors, then restore the canine and premolar areas with side-by-side implants. This would have been not only a functional compromise but an esthetic one as well. A much better choice would have been to move the canines back into their correct positions, leaving a site for a lateral incisor implant mesial to each canine and a premolar implant to the to the distal; thus the canine would be unrestored and in an ideal position for proper canine disclusion. As is almost always the case, the result was better and easier to achieve functionally and esthetically.

Chapter 11

Experiments Regarding the Stability of Implant Materials

1. Gainesforth & Higley (1945) [11] used titanium screws for orthodontic anchorage in six dogs. These implants were inserted in the ramus area and immediately attached to a device designed to retract the maxillary cuspids. All the screws are lost within 16-31 days.

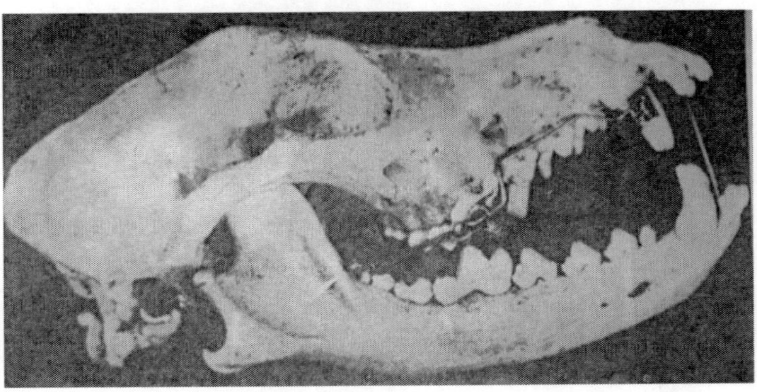

Figure 19. Cuspid retraction with the help of Implants in dog.

2. Sherman (1978) [12] inserted vitreous Carbon implants in 6 dogs in the 3rd premolar are. The implants were allowed to heal for 70 days before being loaded with 175 gms of force. After 2 weeks only 2 implants were stable. But other studies confirmed that vitreous carbon implants resist movement if allowed to heal before being loaded with forces upto 200 gms for as long as 7 months.

3. Smith (1979) [13] evaluated two stage bioglass coated Aluminium oxide implants which were placed in mandibular molars in monkeys. After 12 weeks healing period, the bilateral mandibular implants were loaded with 425 gms of continuous force for 2-9 weeks. The implants remained stationary except for a slight movement of 0.3 mm when the force was doubled.
4. Eugene Roberts (1984) [16] inserted pure titanium screw shaped implant into the femur of the rabbits, after healing for 6-12 weeks the paired implants were loaded with 100 gms of force for 1-12 weeks. Histologically there was an increase in bone mass at area of loading.
5. Roberts (1989) [19] conducted a study on dog mandibles and found that 10% bone contact was sufficient enough to resist loads. An endosseous implant inadvertently penetrated the periodontal ligament and part of the root of a mandibular canine which showed histologic signs of normal healing.

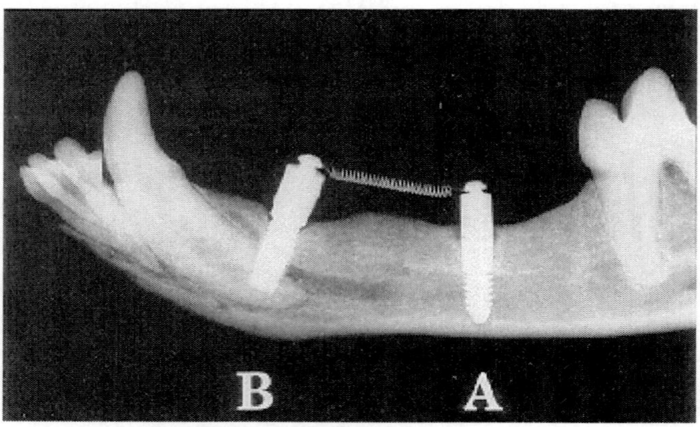

Figure 20. Implant placed in dog mandible showing excellent healing.

Chapter 12

Clinical Uses of Implants in Orthodontics

Anchorage

Implants offer to solve one of the orthodontists greatest dilemmas that is anchorage control. When teeth are used for anchorage purpose they experience a reciprocal effect by the forces applied by he remaining teeth to move to their desired positions especially in case of critical anchorage. The reciprocal nature of forces can be avoided by the innate stability of an osseointegrated implant device as the implants are rigidly embedded in bone they offer a good stability as a source of anchorage.

Differences between prosthetic implants and implants used for orthodontic purpose:

1. Prosthetic implant is stressed with intense interrupted forces directed along the long axis
2. Orthodontic implant need to resist less intense but continuous forces that are perpendicular to its long axis

Key to implant stability is the lack of a complete fibrous capsule. If a complete capsule or pseudoperiodontal ligament were to exist the implant would react to all orthodontic force similar to a tooth.

Anchorage Purpose

Orthopedic – Maxillary expansion.
Maxillary Protraction.
Orthodontic – Intrusion, space closure, Distalization.

Orthopaedic Use

Maxillary Expansion

Ankylosis of a tooth is usually a major problem for the orthodontist. Occasionally this immobility can be useful.

Guyman et al. (1980) [14] intentionally ankylosed maxillary permanent Lateral incisors in three monkeys to act as pseudoimplants. He extracted the lateral incisors, curetted the sockets and replanted the endodontically treated teeth over an hour later. By 8 weeks, the lateral incisors demonstrated the classical signs of ankylosis.

An expansion device was attached to the ankylosed teeth and forces of 1-2 pounds caused no tooth movement, palatal widening occurred by skeletal expansion. As often occurs with reimplanted teeth, however there was widespread root resorption noted on all aspects of the lateral incisors.

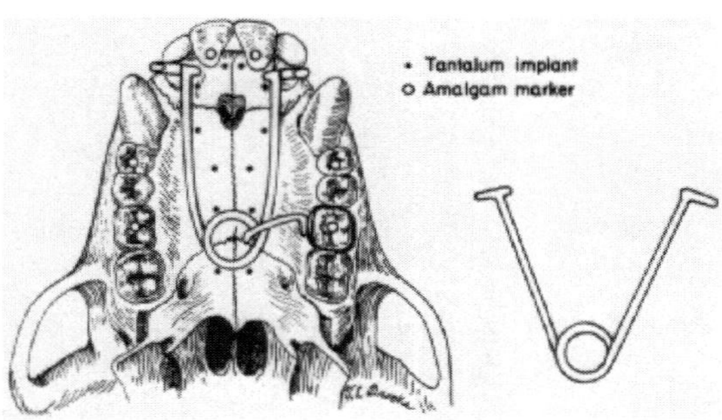

Figure 21. Ankylosed lateral incisors with expansion device in monkey.

Movassaghi (1995) [84] investigated the ability to use titanium screws to provide stable skeletal points in the growing craniofacial region of the rabbit for suture expansion. These screws provided sites for direct application of external forces to alter growth and anatomic form.

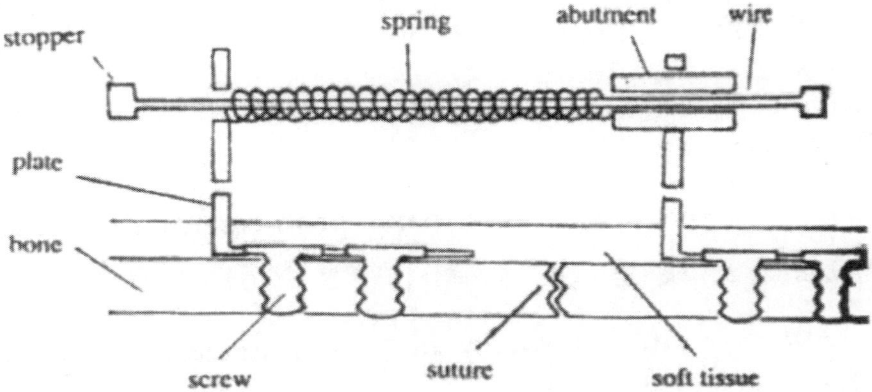

Figure 22. Expansion device with titanium screws in rabbit.

These pure titanium craniofacial plates were contoured into 'L' shape with a 90° angle at the midpoint. The plates were placed bilaterally in the frontal and nasal bone sites and had a diameter of 2 mm and length of 4mm. After 4 weeks of healing a spring mechanism with a distraction force of 55 gms was activated between ipsilateral plates and across the fronto nasal sutures bilaterally and a significant increase in growth about 6 mm was seen across the fronto nasal suture.

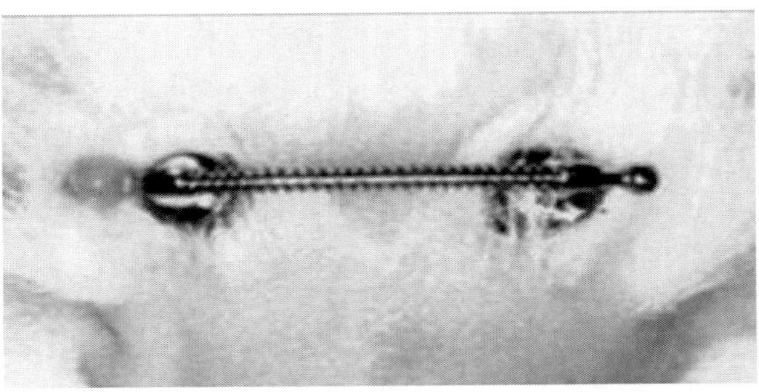

Figure 23. Appliance used to provide expansion load to suture. An open coil spring has been compressed between the abutments to provide the expansion load. An .040 ball clasp has been used to hold the spring in place between abutments. Light cure resin ensures the ball clasp does not disengage the abutments.

Parr et al. (1997) [23] conducted experiments on sutural expansion using rigidly integrated endosseous implants. As they offer great advantage for orthodontic and orthopedic anchorage in the oral and midfacial regions. To evaluate the use of endosseous implants in the mid face region 2 flanged titanium implants were placed on either side of the midnasal suture of rabbits – they were divided into 2 groups. For one group the force was applied was 1 N and the other group was 3 N. All implants remained stable during the loading. The distance between the implants increased significantly in the loaded groups and was higher in 3 N group.

Multiple Fluorochrome Images

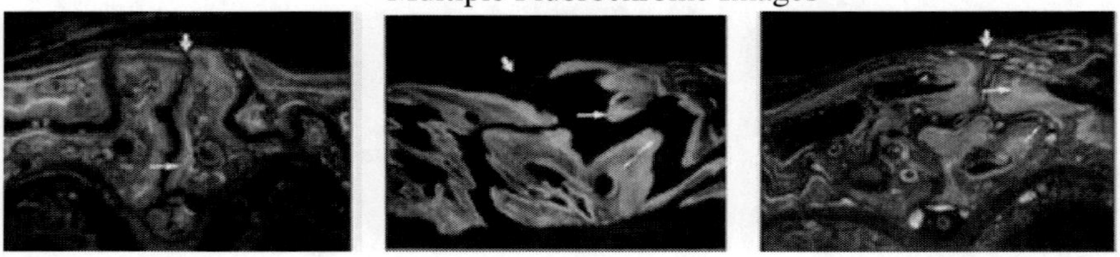

(a) (b) (c)

Figure 24. Fluorochrome images of nasal suture (a) Unloaded control Horizontal arrows mark sharp label due to lamellar bone formation (b-c) Loaded implants leading to expansion of nasal suture. Horizontal arrows mark diffuse label due to woven bone formation.

Maxillary Protraction

The concept of intentional ankylosis was extended to the treatment of a midface deficient juvenile with Apert anomaly by Shapiro & Kokich [85] in 1985. a protraction headgear was attached to deciduous maxillary cuspids to protract the maxilla which was effective. But the main disadvantage is the probability that the ankylosed cuspid may destabilize from root resorption before treatment is complete.

Smalley et al. (1988) [17] demonstrated the potential of implants for orthopaedic movements. They placed Branemark implants into the maxilla, zygoma and orbital and occipital bones of 4 monkeys using an external protraction device attached to the orbital and occipital implants, a constant force of 600 gms/side was applied to the maxillary or zygomatic bones for 12-18 weeks.

They demonstrated a 12mm widening of the zygomaticomaxillary suture and 16 mm of zygomaticotemporal sutures a change from Class I to a Class II dental relationship and increase in overjet of 5 to 7 mm. The facial implants remained immobile throughout the experiment.

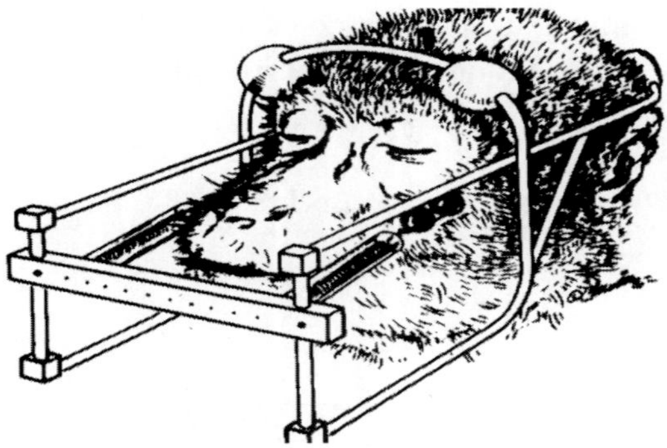

Figure 25. The framework is rigidly attached with self-curing acrylic resin to the four cranial titanium implants. A precision coil spring with a protective tube was fastened bilaterally from the adjustable anterior horizontal bar of the framework to the facial titanium implants.

All the above uses of implants i.e., for orthopaedic purpose are best effective in growing individuals in whom active growth due to remodeling changes is occurring.

Implants for Space Closure

Use of Endosseous Implant for Closure of Extraction Space or Protraction of Molar

Eugene Roberts (1994) [86] used an endosseous implants in the retro molar region as an anchorage for closing the atrophic extraction site in the region of lower left 1st molar.

This patient has FPD in the region of lower left 1st molar with extruded and mesially tipped 2nd molar abutment. The patient wanted to remove the bridge and close the extraction space. Treatment options were

1. To place an implant
2. To replace the 1st molar (By autotransplantation of 3rd molar. This was ruled out because of poor residual ridge and apical foramen of 3rd molar was already closed)
3. Close the extraction space by using reverse pull headgear. This was ruled out because
    a. It is difficult to apply a unilateral protraction force

b. It is difficult to apply the countermoment for translation.
c. It is difficult to apply the intrusion force on already extruded 3rd molar

So therefore it was decided to use implant in the retromolar region for anchorage purpose.

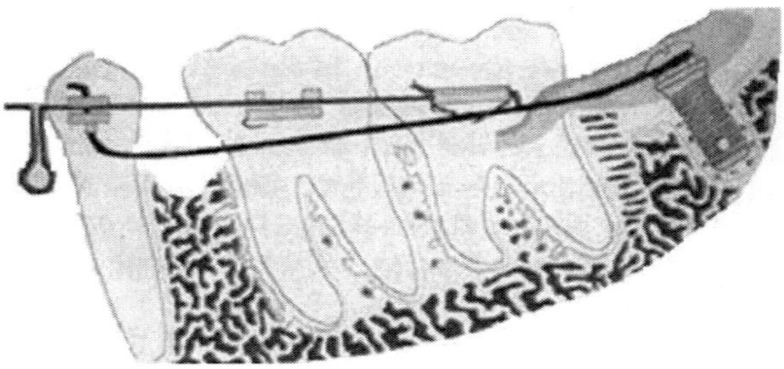

Figure 26. Endosseous Implant in retromolar region for space closure.

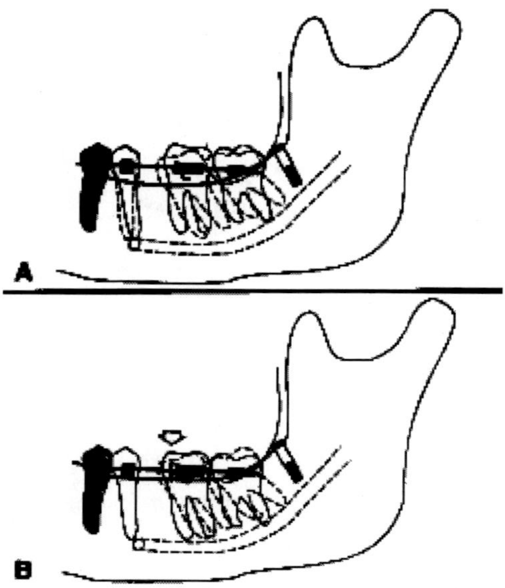

Figure 27. Endosseous Implant in retromolar region for space. Closure: (A) Levelling and aligning stage (B) Posterior molar intrusion using the implant for vertical anchorage.

For this purpose a 0.022 slot PEA was used and endosseous implant was placed in the retromolar region. After the initial leveling and aligning the 3rd molar was intruded using retromolar implant for vertical anchorage. A sectional archwire was attached to the implant at one end and hooked on to main archwire in the premolar region. This sectional archwire was shaped on to 3rd molar to apply the intrusive force.

Then upper/lower 19x25 archwires with a keyhole loop was fabricated. Protraction of lower molars was achieved by applying both lingual and buccal mesializing force. The buccal force was applied by activation of closing loop. The lingual force was applied by lingual arch which was placed 3 mm mesial to the 2nd molar and forcefully engaged into the lingual sheath. Now the retraction of the premolar was avoided by connecting the 2nd premolar to the retromolar implant with a rigid wire.

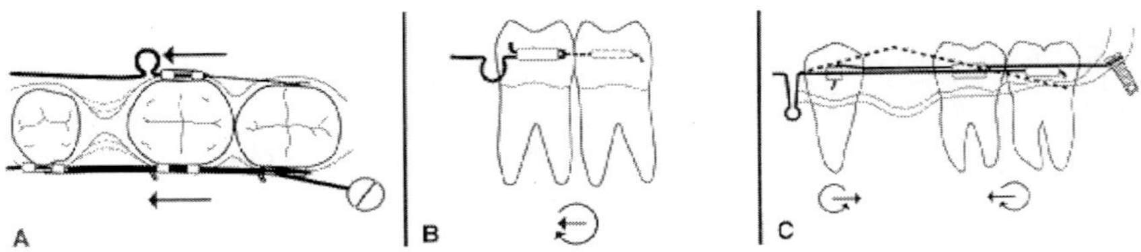

Figure 28. Endosseous Implant in retromolar region for space. Closure: (A) Space closure using closing loop in 19X25 archwire (B) Clockwise moment on molars (C) Clockwise and anticlockwise moments on anterior and posterior segment respectively during space closure.

Skeletal Anchorage System – For Open Bite Correction

Sugauwara; Umemori et al. (1999) [87]. Use of implants for open bite correction is described by *Sugawara and Umemori*. They called this method as *Skeletal Anchorage System (SAS)*. Control of vertical dimensions is very important in correction of anterior open bite. Use of multiband bracketed appliance, extraoral anchorage, magnets and vertical chin cup are not effective in achieving molar intrusion for correction of anterior open bite especially in adult patients. This is because it is difficult to attain rigid anchorage for molar extrusion with the above mentioned methods. So the author developed skeletal anchorage system using Titanium plates as a source of anchorage for intruding the molars.

The implants used are 'L' shaped Titanium implants.

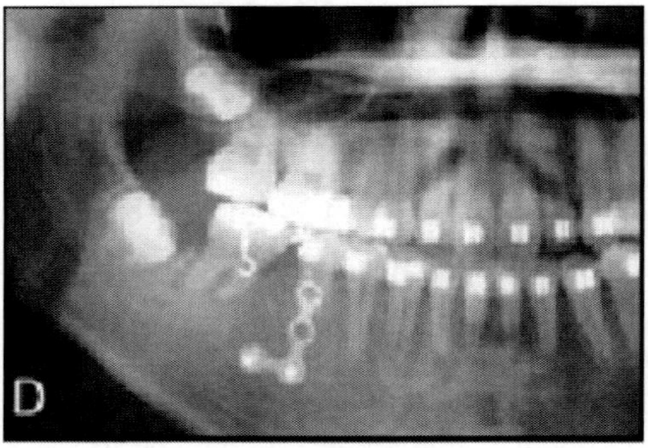

Figure 29. Radiograph showing 'L' shaped titanium implant for molar intrusion in open bite cases.

Surgical procedure: Done under LA. A mucoperiosteal flap is raised in the apical region of the 1st or 2nd molar and the cortical bone is exposed. The 'L' shaped miniplate is adjusted to fit the contour of the cortical bone and fixed to the bone by using screws, with long arm exposed to the oral cavity. Then wait till the wound healing occurs and elastic force was applied from molar to the miniplate for intrusion. Lingual crown torque was applied in the lingual arch to prevent the buccal flaring as the molar intrudes and after the treatment the miniplates are removed.

Skeletal Anchorage System (For Deep Bite Correction)

Creekmore; Eklund et al. (1983) [88] inserted a surgical vitallium bone screw just below anterior nasal spine.

Ten days after the screw was placed, a light elastic thread was tied from the head of the screw to the archwire. The elastic thread was renewed throughout treatment, so that a continous force was maintained 24 hrs a day. After 1 year they found that the maxillary central incisors were elevated 6mms and torqued lingually about 25 degrees.

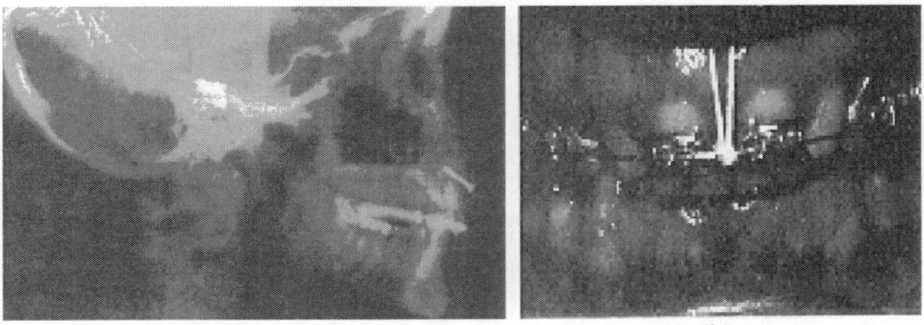

(a) (b)

Figure 30. Radiograph of surgical vitallium bone screw below anterior nasal spine (a) Lateral view (b) Frontal view.

Impacted Titanium Post

Though endosseous implants will provide a good source of anchorage, the procedure of placing and removing them is very difficult. Impacted titanium provides a simple alternative as a source of anchorage.

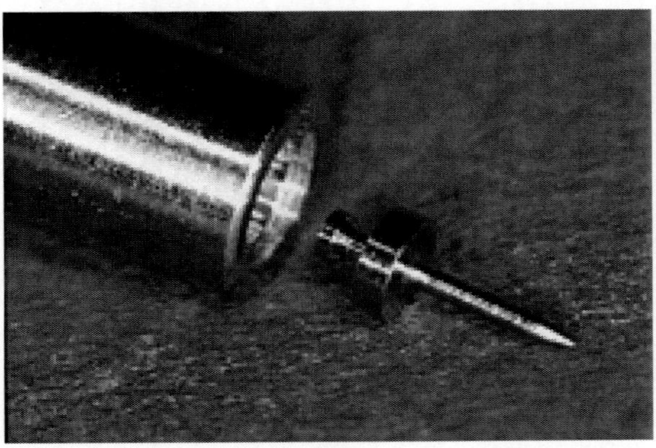

Figure 31-1. Titanium post with mechanical impactor.

Boussquet et al. (1996) [89] used impacted titanium post for retraction of 1st premolar in upper 2nd premolar extraction case. The impacted Ti was used as an anchorage on right side while on left side 1st premolar was retracted conventionally serving as a means of control. Ti Post: of 6 mm in length and 0.7mm diameter was used. The instrument called mechanical impactor was used to place the post. Then the Ti post was placed between the 1st molar and extraction site of 2nd premolar. Four weeks of healing is allowed. Then complete strap up is done. After this the right first molar is connected to Ti post with 0.040 wire. The upper 1st molars are connected by TPA made of 0.032” ss wire.

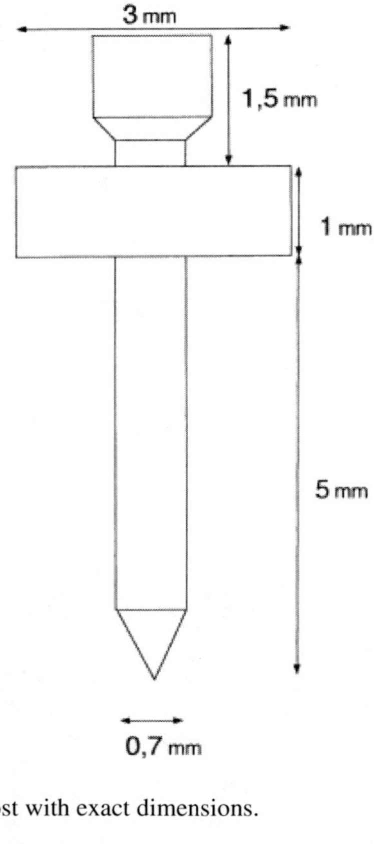

Figure 31-2. Titanium post with exact dimensions.

Unlike a conventional TPA this is attached on facial side and then an offset is placed. The TPA traverses the anterior segment again on the other side mesial to the molar an offset is placed. An acrylic splint is used to join to the TP wire in the incisors.

The mesial movement of molar is assessed by the marks drawn on the TPA wires at the molar tube. Then the premolars are retracted by sectional 16* 16 archwire.After 3 months the impacted post was intact in its position and right side PM retraction was complete without anchorage loss but on the left side PM retraction was completed with some anchor loss.

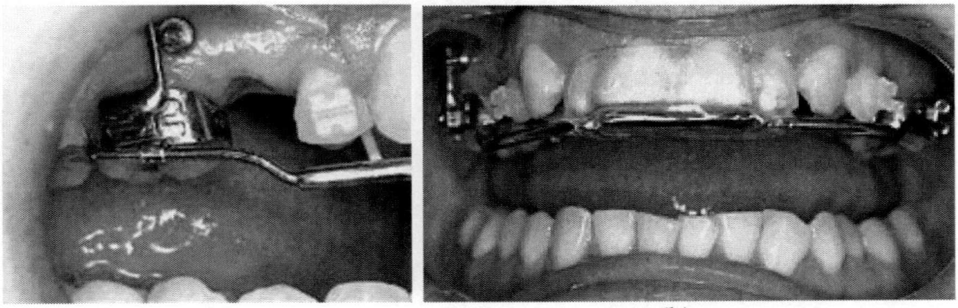

(a) (b)

Figure 31-3. Titanium post with TPA Intraoral View (a) Right buccal view (b) Frontal view.

The Reconstruction of Bilateral Clefts using Endosseous Implants after Bone Grafting

Hiroaki et al. (2002) [90] carried out the orthodontic reconstruction of an adult bilateral cleft patient with a severe Class III malocclusion in which endosseous implants were inserted after secondary alveolar bone grafting. The patient was a 21-year-old Japanese male whose lateral incisors were congenitally missing and whose premaxilla was inclined lingually. The occlusion was classified as Angle Class III with an overjet of 8 mm. Orthodontic alignment was initiated to correct the position of the maxillary incisors before bone grafting. After the anterior occlusal relationship was corrected, bilateral alveolar clefts were reconstructed by bone grafting with autogenous particulate marrow and cancellous bone harvested from the iliac crest. ITI-SLA fixtures (Institute Straumann, Waldenburg, Switzerland) (length, 10 mm; diameter, 4.1 mm) were placed into the grafted bonefor prosthetic restoration of the missing lateral incisors. The results illustrate that this protocol can be expected to provide an acceptable occlusion and good dentoalveolar stability in adult cleft patients.

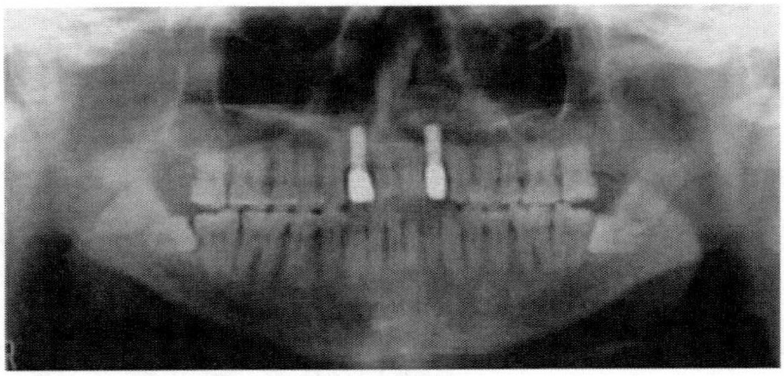

(a)

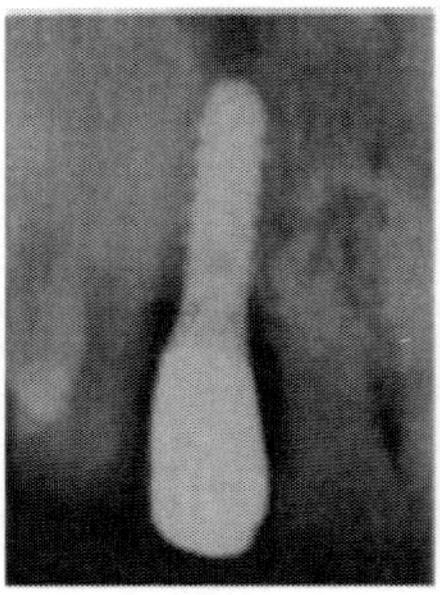

(b)

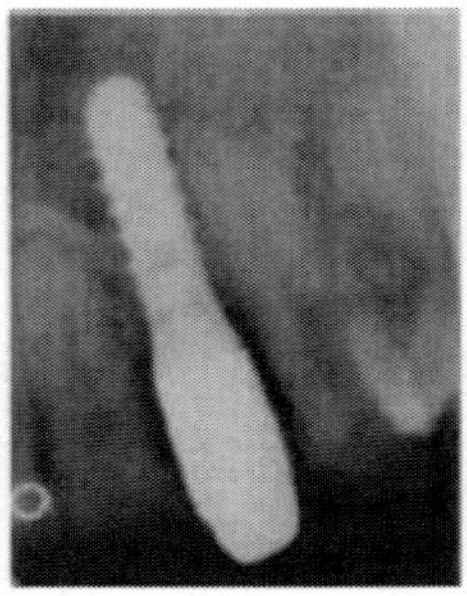

(c)

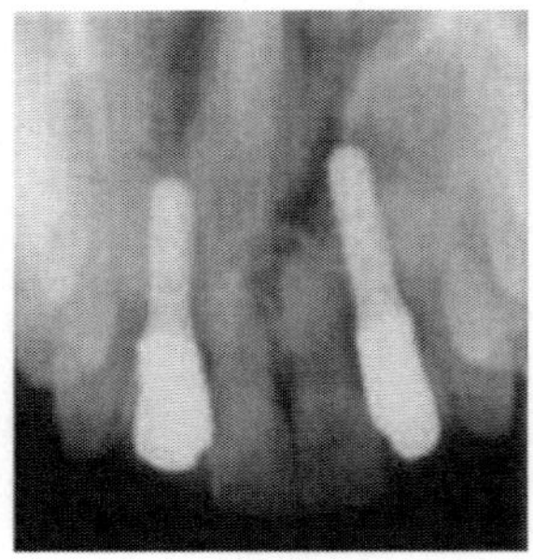

(d)

Figure 31-4. Radiographic views of Endosseous Implants (a) OPG (b) Rt. Lateral IOPA (c) Lt. Lateral IOPA (d) Frontal IOPA.

Chapter 13

Newer Implant Systems

Endosseous implants have following disadvantages

1. Invasive surgical procedure
2. Long healing period
3. Cost factor

The ongoing research related to use of implants in orthodontics was focused on developing an implant which is relatively simpler to use. In these series are included

1. Mini-implant
2. Onplant
3. Orthoimplant
4. Modular Transitional Implant (MTI)
5. Microimplant

Mini-implant: Ryuzo kanomi (1997) [91]. Conventional implants are cumbersome to the patient because of the surgery and discomfort during healing. For orthodontic anchorage, the implant should besuch that it can be placed in any area, and the surgical procedure should be simple so that an orthodontist or general dentist can do it. The removal of the implant should be easy after it's use is over. To meet the above requirements Ryuzo Kanomi (1997) [97] used an implant made of miniscrews to fix the bone plates. This mini-implant was *1.2mm in diameter, 6mm long.*

Surgical Procedure

Under local anesthesia, a mini-bone screw was implanted in the alveolar bone between the root apices of the mandibular central incisors.

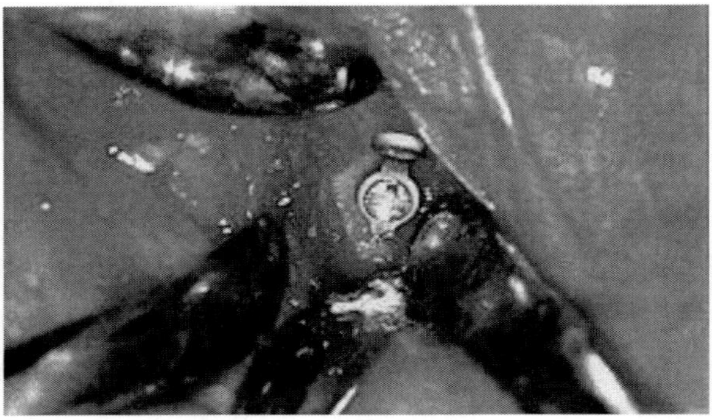

Figure 32. Mini-implant placed intraorally.

Three additional screws were implanted, under the root alveolus of the maxillary central incisor and on both sides of the missing mandibular second premolar, for future traction. Each implant was placed 2-3mm from the root apex. The implant procedure was as follows:

1. Open a mucoperiosteal flap and denude the alveolar bone. Drill into the cortical bone with a 2mm round bur, using water cooling, to make a pit about 1.5mm in diameter.

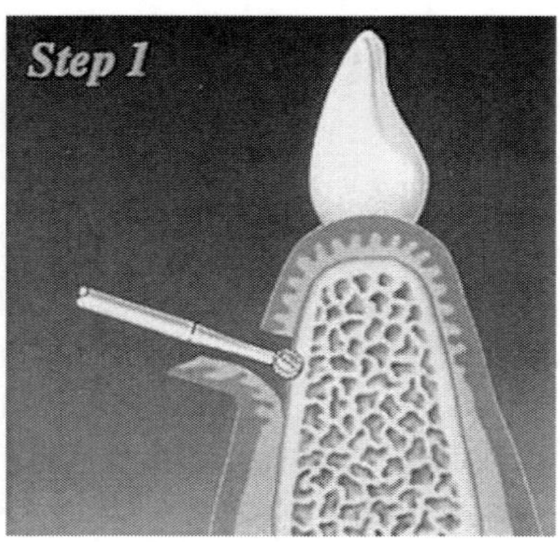

Figure 33. Drilling of pit in alveolar bone with round bur.

2. Drill into the bone with a 1mm pilot drill, still using water cooling, as far as the length of the mini-implant.

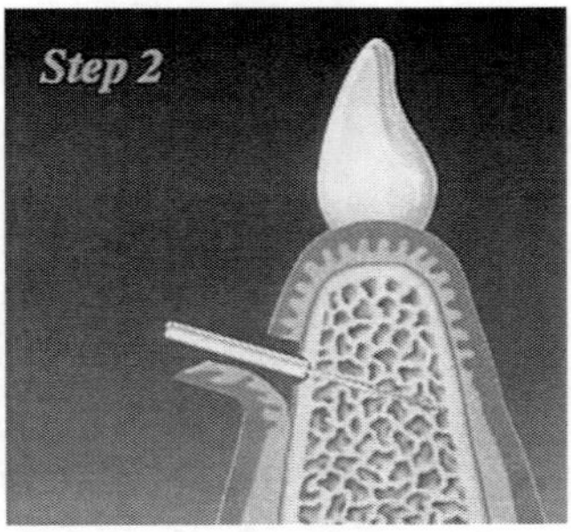

Figure 34. Drilling in alveolar bone with pilot drill.

3. Insert the implant with the accompanying miniature screwdriver.

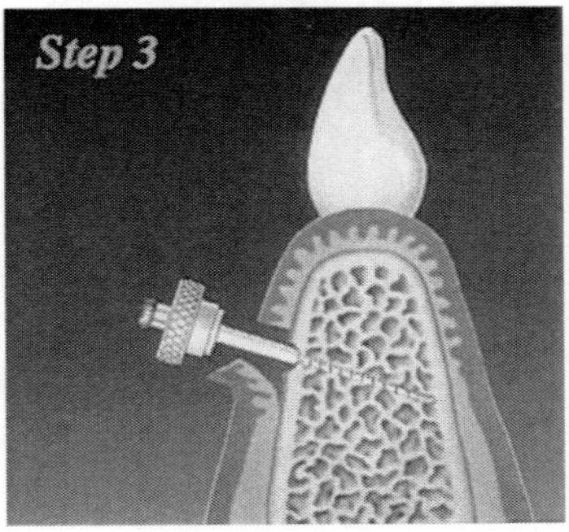

Figure 35. Insertion of Implant using screwdriver.

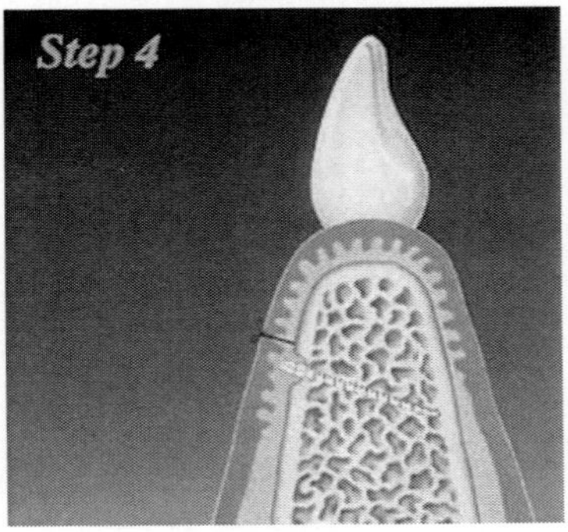

Figure 36. Implant covered with flap and sutured.

4. Cover the implant with the flap, and suture the wound. Document the position of the implant with a periapical x-ray.
5. After healing and osseointegration, remove the gingival tissue covering the mini-implant.

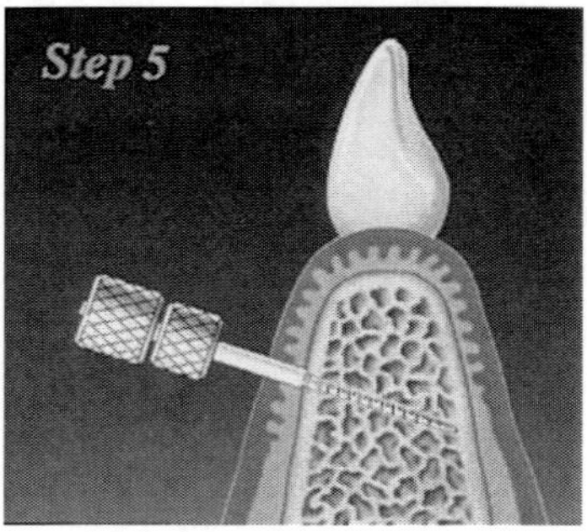

Figure 37. Removal of gingival tissue around mini-implant.

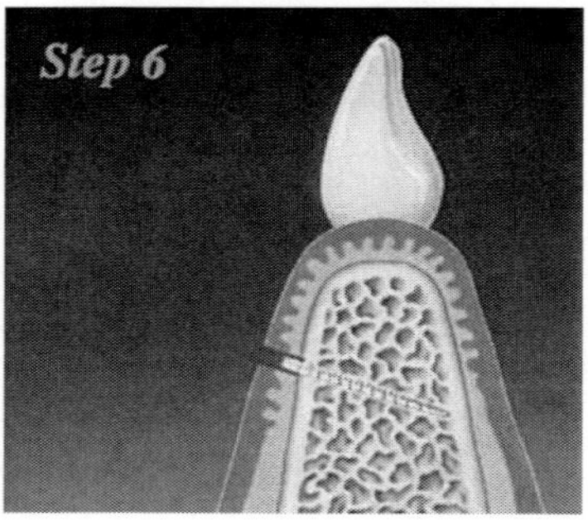

Figure 38. Removal of soft tissue around mini-implant with mucosal punch.

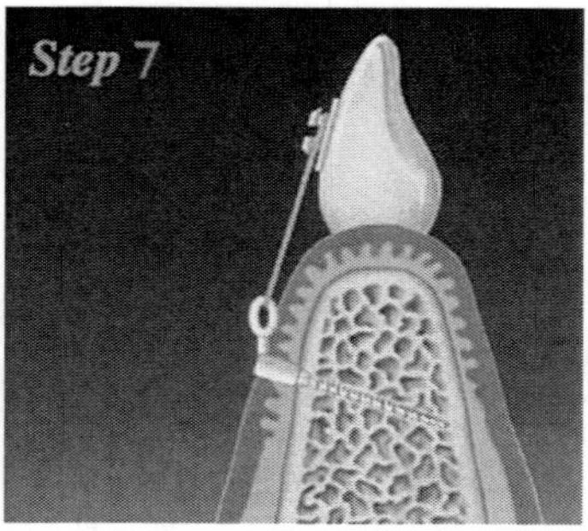

Figure 39. Attacment of a two-hole titanium bone plate to the head of the mini-implant to act as a hook.

6. Using a mucosal punch, remove the soft tissue surrounding the head of the mini-implant.
7. Attach a two-hole titanium bone plate to the head of the mini-implant to act as a hook.

Tie a ligature wire or elastic chain between this hook and the bracket on the tooth or teeth to be intruded—in this case, the mandibular central incisors.

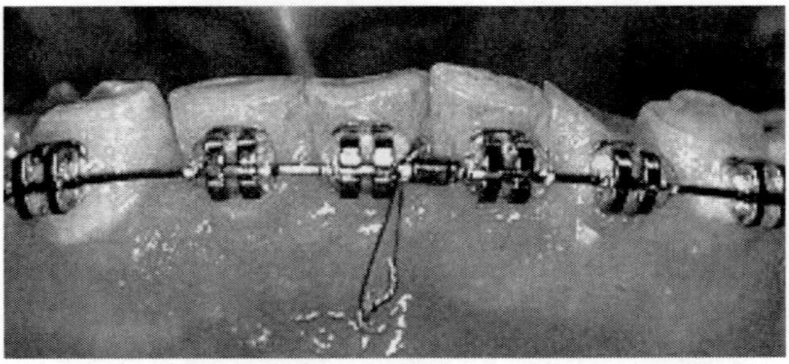

Figure 40. Attachment of a ligature wire to the hook of the implant and the bracket/archwire to intrude the lower incisors.

Onplant and Orthoimplant

Though conventional osseointegrated implants are best means of anchorage control, their disadvantage is their removal after orthodontic treatment is very difficult. The recent forms of implants (ie) OnPlant and orthoimplant overcome this problem. Their removal after the use is relatively easier.

OnPlant

This was given by *Block & Hoffman* (2000) [92].

The OnPlant, which resembles a button, is a relatively flat, disc-shaped fixture available in diameters of 8mm and 10mm. It has a textured, hydroxyapatite-coated surface for integration with the palatal bone.

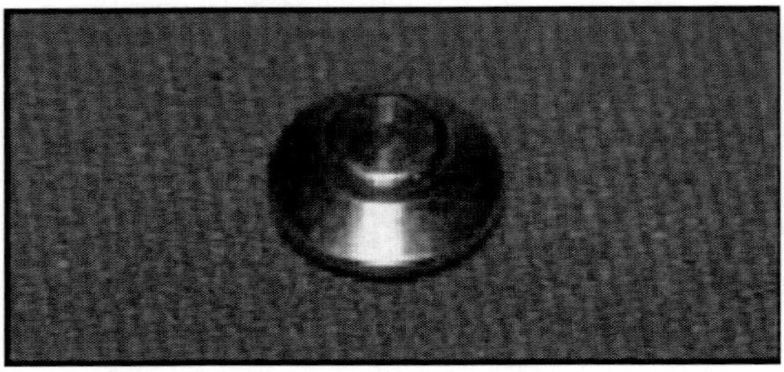

Figure 41. Onplant.

Surgical placement involves making an incision in the palatal mucosa outward from the midline. The tissue is tunneled under, in full-thickness fashion, past the midline to the eventual implantation site.

The OnPlant is then slipped under the soft tissue and brought into position, and the incision is sutured.

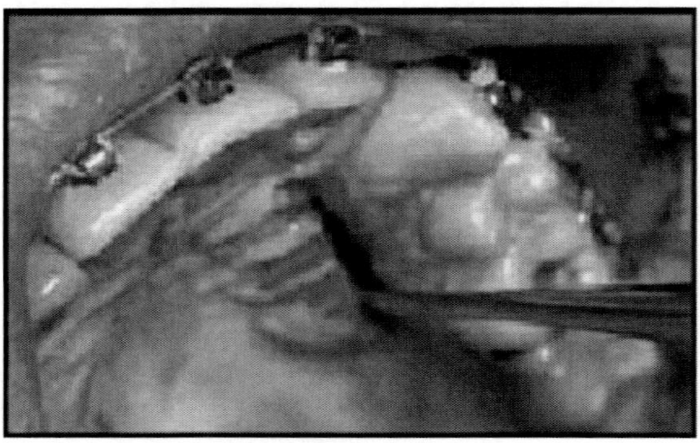

Figure 42. Incision in the palatal mucosa outward from the midline.

A vacuformed stent is worn for 10 days to place pressure on the OnPlant. This step is crucial to the device's integration, which takes at least four months. Once integration has been achieved, an open-tray impression is taken by exposing the OnPlant, removing its cover screw, and securing an impression coping. A simulated implant is used to pour the working cast.

A transpalatal arch is attached to the OnPlant and bonded or banded to the teeth on both sides of the arch. When the OnPlant is no longer needed for anchorage, it is explanted by soft-tissue exposure and de-integrated with a carefully aimed chisel.

The OnPlant is a relatively easy device to place, secure and can be removed. However, it should be noted that this is not an endosseous implant;

since it lies superficial to the bone, it should be considered a subperiosteal implant.

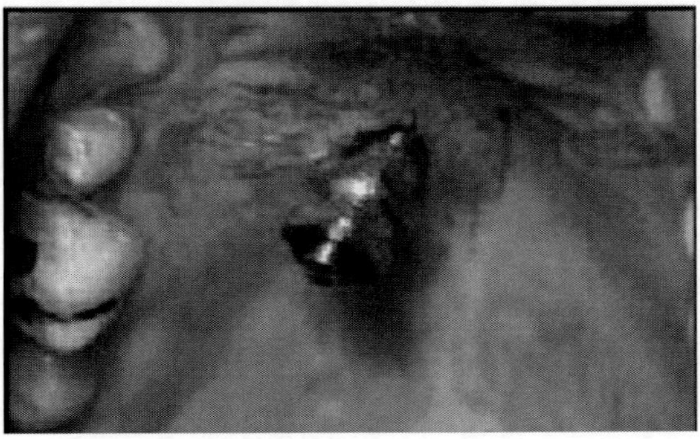

Figure 43. Onplant placed.

Additional Studies Involving the OnPlant Device [79]

Molar distalization: An OnPlant was placed mid-palatally opposite the maxillary second premolars. The maxillary third molars were extracted bilaterally. The right and left maxillary second molars were prepared for full-crown cast restorations, which were soldered to a rigid transpalatal bar. An expansion device was soldered to the transpalatal bar and secured to the abutment using a cast attachment.

The spring expansion device was activated to provide 150 to 200 g of continuous distal force to the second molars. The cast crowns and rigid transpalatal bar ensured bodily movement. The second molars were bodily distalized 6.0 mm in 11 months. The OnPlant device remained stationary and did not migrate in reference to the remaining teeth in the maxilla. After sacrifice, the tissues were removed, demonstrating the bodily distalization of the maxillary second molar anchored only by the OnPlant device.

Tooth movements of this type are not easily achieved. The orthodontist may use the OnPlant to anchor distalising forces, thus expanding treatment choices when dealing with maxillary dental protrusion, crowding, or Class II malocclusion.

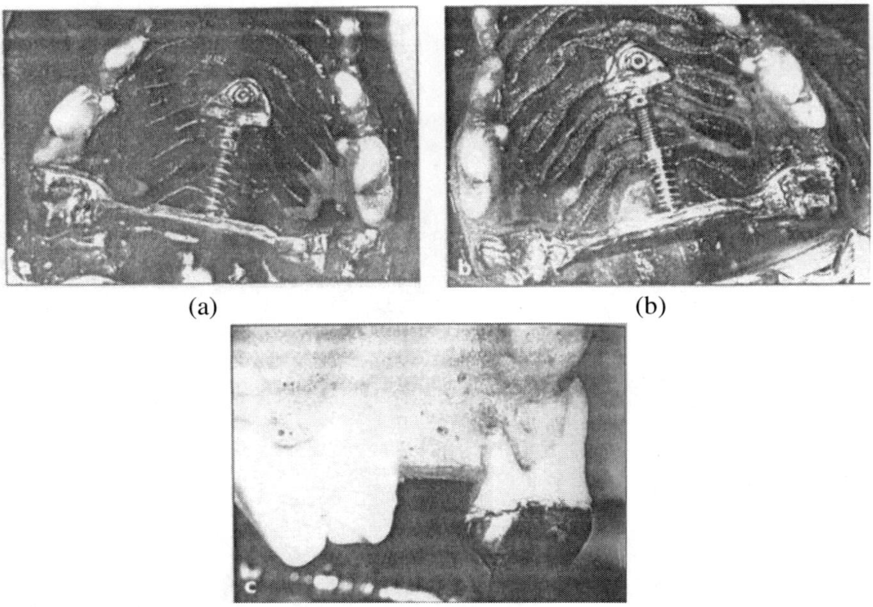

(a) (b)

(c)

Figure 44. Onplant placed for molar distalization (a) Transpalatal arch attached to the Onplant with screw (b) Activated screw with molar distalization via TPA (c) Buccal view of space created by the distalized molar.

Mandibular Lengthening Using OnPlants to Anchor the Distraction Device

Block and Zoldes (unpublished data) used two OnPlant devices unilaterally positioned on the lateral surface of a dog's mandible to anchor a distraction device. This was the first use of an intraoral device anchored by on-plants to the mandible to distract the mandible and lengthen its corpus.

The OnPlants were placed against the mandibular body after creation of a subperiosteai tunnel originating from the alveolar crest.

In the laboratory, a custom-cast L-shaped attachment was made to attach to the OnPlant by a screw into a prosthetic abutment. The vertical component of the custom attachment engaged the jaws of a small Howmedica mini-lengthener. At the time of creation of the osteotomy, the attachment was placed after the lateral aspect of the mandible was exposed.

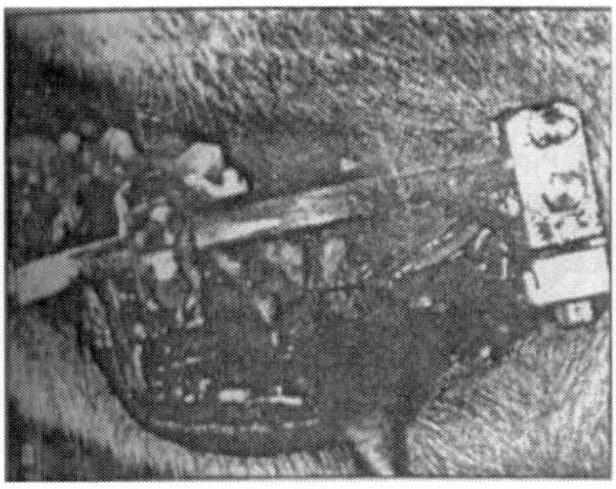

(a)

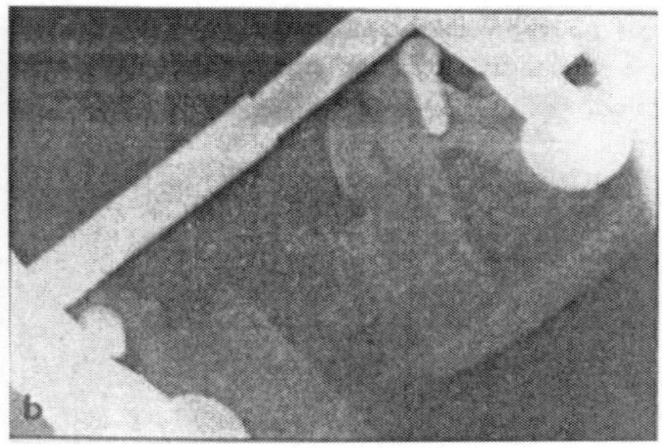

(b)

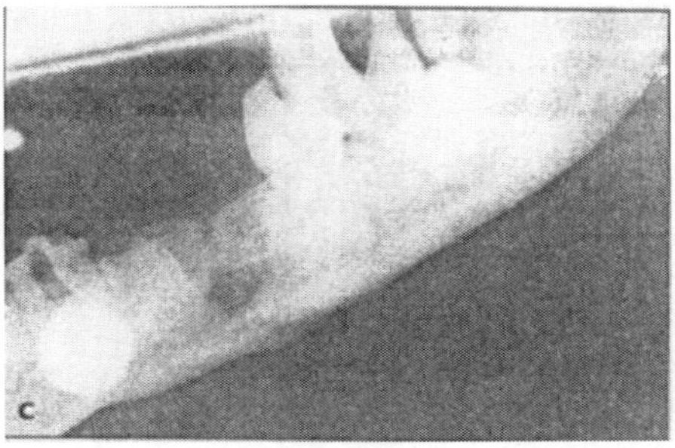

(c)

Figure 45. Onplant for mandibular distraction in dog's mandible (a) Distraction device placed in the mandible anchored to Onplant (b) Radiograph showing activated device with mandibular lengthening (c) Onplants still in place as the bone forms at the distraction site.

After approximately 12 weeks for integration of the OnPlant. an incision was made on the crest and a split-thickness dissection was achieved. The healing screws of the OnPlants were removed and replaced by prosthetic abutments, and the custom-cast L-shaped attachment was placed. A bur was used to create a corticotomy along the buccal cortex, full thickness above and inferior to the inferior alveolar nerve canal. The lingual plate was gently fractured, preserving the integrity of the neurovascular bundle. The previously adjusted mini-lengthener was positioned. After 7 days for healing, distraction was accomplished 0.5 mm twice a day for 10 consecutive days, for a total of 10 mm of unilateral elongation. The inferior alveolar nerve was monitored throughout the experiment by the use of a jaw-jerk reflex without loss of nerve function. Radiographic evidence of bone formation within the distraction gap was present at 6 weeks.

The OnPlant is a device that can use any bone surface as the location of the anchor.

Clinical Field Testing of OnPlants [79]

Four women participated in a pilot field evaluation using prototype devices. They were wearing orthodontic appliances, a headgear (albeit reluctantly), and had critical anchorage requirements, and they welcomed an alternative form of treatment. A single OnPlant was surgically inserted subperiosteally in the midpalatal region. After 4 months, the OnPlant was exposed and a grooved abutment was inserted. Stainless steel bands were fitted to the maxillary first molars, and a polyvinylsiloxane impression technique was used to transfer the bands and abutment location to a vorking cast. A 0.051-inch stainless steel wire rested against the posterior surface of the abutment and was soldered to the bands.

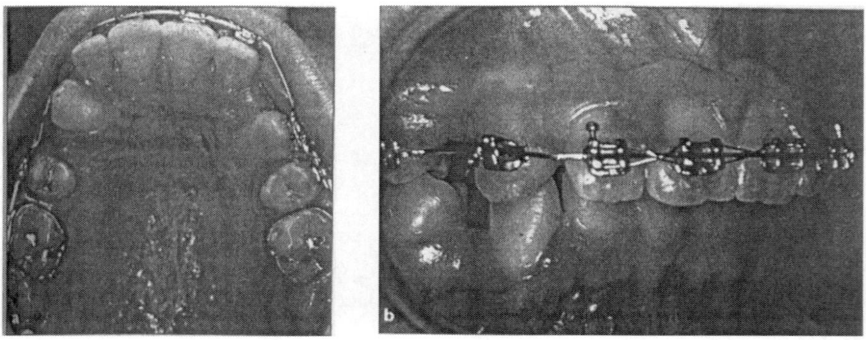

(a) (b)

Figure 46. Anterior Retraction with Onplants (a) Occlusal View (b) Rt. Buccal view.

The anterior maxillary teeth were bodily retracted as a unit, without the aid of elastics or headgear. The OnPlant provided the sole means of anchorage for the dental movements. After the anterior teeth had been retracted into their new positions, the transpalatal wire and the OnPlants were removed. Removal of the OnPlants required local anesthesia, a small incision on the anterior 120 degrees of the OnPlant's circumference, and a periostea! elevator to separate the OnPlant from the palatal bone. The underlying bone had developed a textured pattern to match the undersurface of the OnPlant. In all four patients the palatal tissues were closed and healed without adverse effects.

It is significant that all six anterior teeth were retracted simultaneously. In many conventional orthodontic treatment schemes, the canines are retracted before the incisors. Theoretically, this technique of "divide and conquer" reduces the strain on the posterior units. These sequential methods create large diastemas between the canines and lateral incisors during conventional treatment, which can be a serious deterrent for prospective patients. Esthetics is a powerful motivational factor in the decision to tolerate orthodontic treatment. Although the spaces are transient, solutions that avoid the problem offer an advantage.

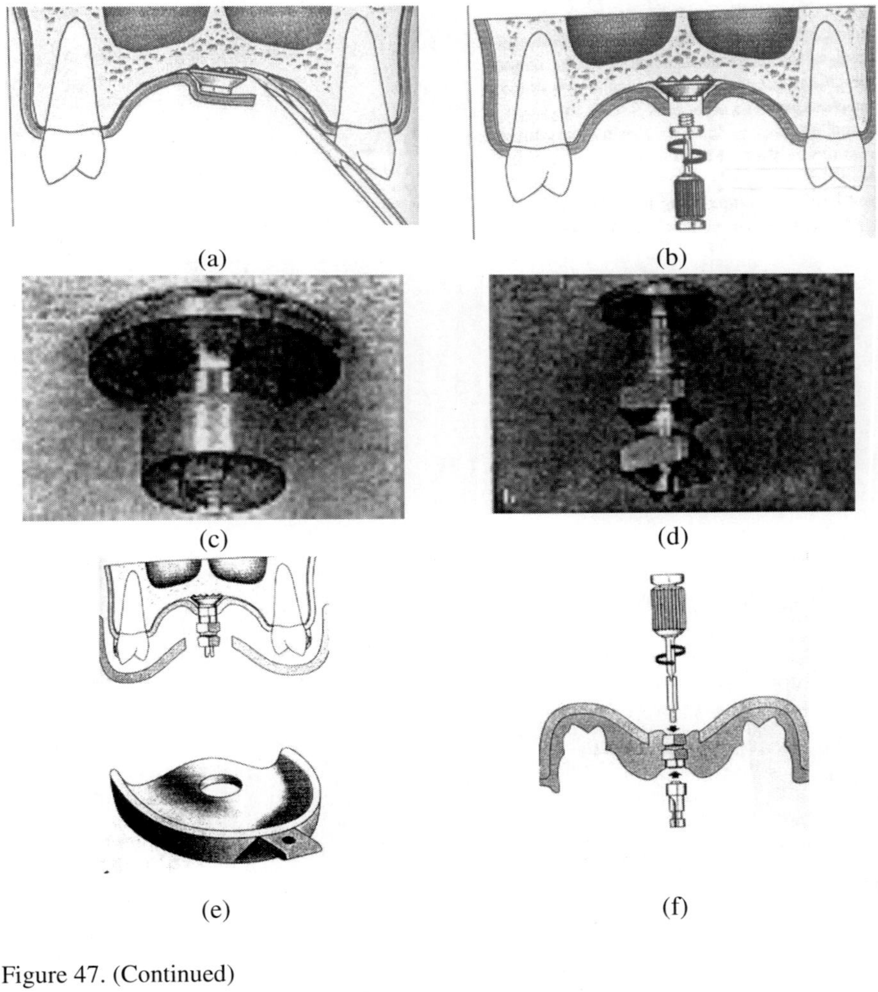

(a) (b) (c) (d) (e) (f)

Figure 47. (Continued)

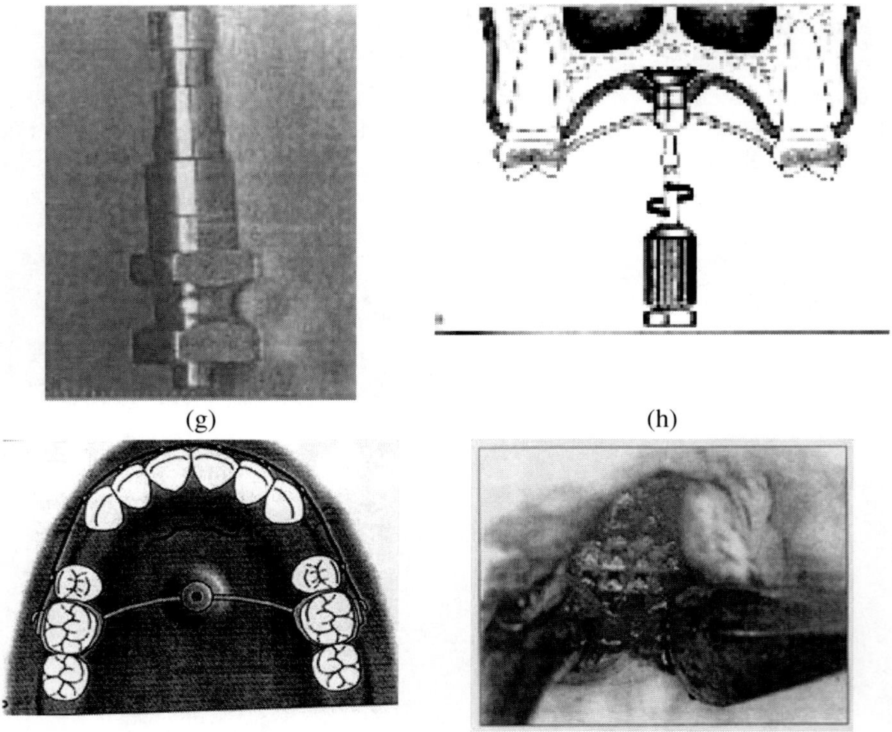

(g) (h)

(i) (j)

Figure 47. Anterior Retraction with Onplants: (a) Placement of the OnPlant through the subperiosteal (b) Removal of the cover screw of the OnPlant tunnel (c) Screw-retained transgingival abutment placed on the external hex of the OnPlant (d) Transfer coping placed in the transgingival abutment (e) After placement of the abutment, the transfer coping is placed and an impression is taken using an open-tray technique. The cast is then poured (f) Onplant analog placed into the transfer coping (g) Onplant analog attached to the transfer coping (h) Abutment with the laser-welded 0.051-inch wire placed on the cast (i) Onplant with transpalatal wire attached to the teeth (j) Texture of the palatal bone, which mirrors the textured surface of the OnPlant.

The implanting and retrieval procedure of the OnPlant was atraumatic. The cost of including the OnPlant therapy can be offset by the reduction in treatment time. Elimination of the compliance factor and control of the result simplify the orthodontist's task, and the hazards of extraoral devices are avoided.

Orthoimplant

This is given by Celenza & Hoffmann (2000) [93].

The Orthoimplant, a true endosseous implant, is an SLA (sandblasted and acid-etched) screw fixture that is inserted into a carefully created osteotomy site in the midpalatal region.

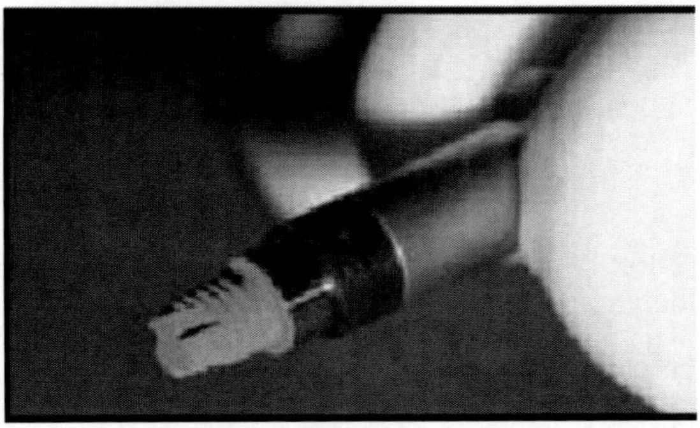

Figure 48. Orthoimplant.

First, an appropriate location must be identified. Next, a soft-tissue trephine is used to remove a small core of palatal mucosa.

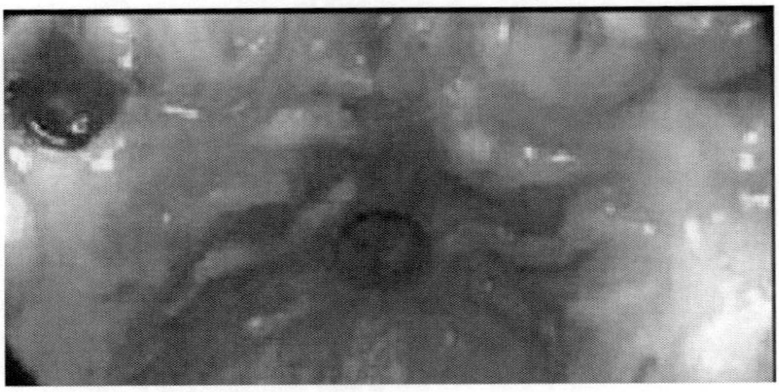

Figure 49. Palatal soft tissue removed.

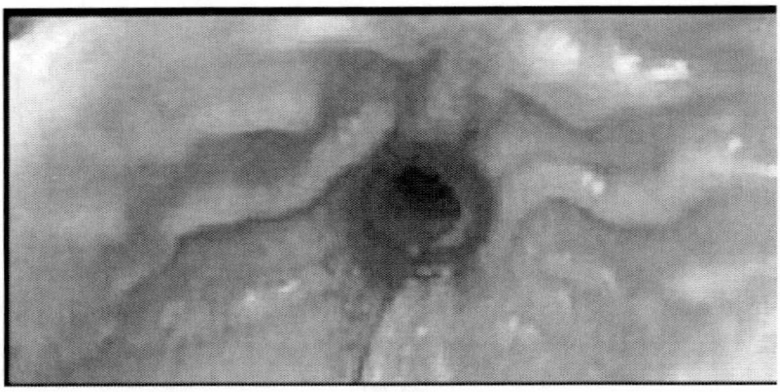

Figure 50. Osteotomy created by round bur.

A round bur then scores the hard palate, followed by a spade adapted to the exact dimensions and proportions of the Orthoimplant. The depth of the osteotomy is either 4mm or 6mm; the outer diameter of the thread is 3.3mm.

The Orthoimplant is screwed into the osteotomy, and a cover screw or cap is placed to control soft tissue overgrowth.

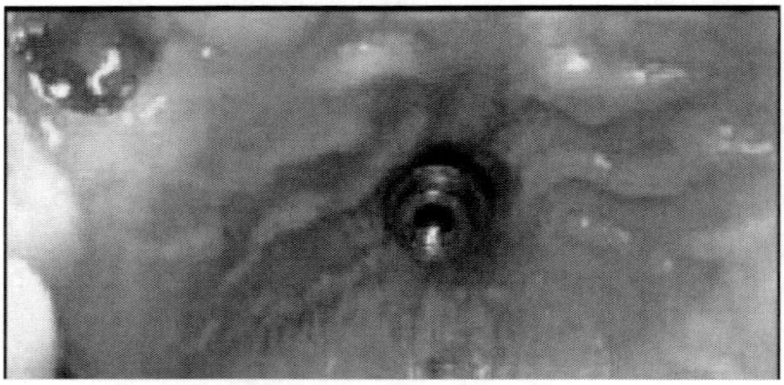

Figure 51. Orthoimplant screwed into the osteotomy site.

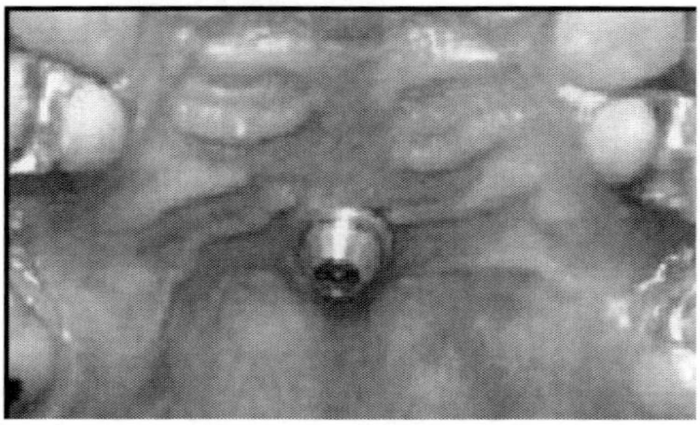

Figure 52. Orthoimplant with Impression Coping.

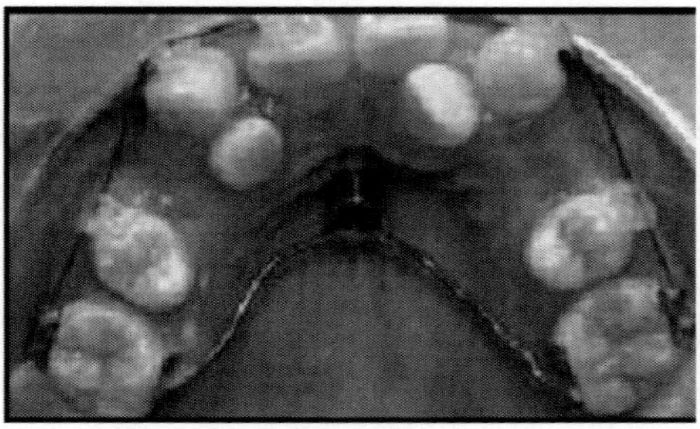

Figure 53. Orthoimplant with Transpalatal Arch.

No suturing is necessary, since a tissue punch was used instead of an incision. After integration has been achieved (in about three months), loading may proceed, although an impression may be taken prior to full integration.

An impression coping is fastened to the Orthoimplant, which greatly facilitates the process and eliminates the need for an open-tray technique.

A transpalatal arch is fastened to the fixture and the desired teeth.

Once the Orthoimplant has accomplished its purpose, it is explanted with a trephine. Healing is usually uneventful.

The Orthoimplant has the advantages of simple placement and utilization. In addition, because it is a true endosseous implant, its integration may be far more predictable than that of the subperiosteal OnPlant.

Microimplant

Park et al. (2001) [94] developed a narrow titanium micro-implant, the Absoanchor, that has a button-shaped head with a hole for ligatures and elastomers. Its small diameter allows its insertion into many areas of the maxilla and mandible that were previously unavailable, such as between the roots of adjacent teeth.

Micro-Implant Selection

The Absoanchor comes in diameters from 1.2mm to 1.6mm for different tasks and sites. Even the smaller 1.2mm and 1.3mm microimplants can withstand as much as 450g of force, whereas most orthodontic applications need forces of less than 300g. The tapered type of micro-implant offers a tighter initial fit than the cylindrical type does, making the first choice for orthodontic use a 1.2mm or 1.3mm tapered micro-implant.

The next larger size should be tried until there is a close fit between screw and bone. A 1.4-1.6mm micro-implant can be used when there is enough space between the roots and greater force is needed.

Serial periapical x-rays should be used to determine whether adequate space exists for implant placement. If enough space is not available, the clinician can consider moving the roots apart orthodontically before placing implants.

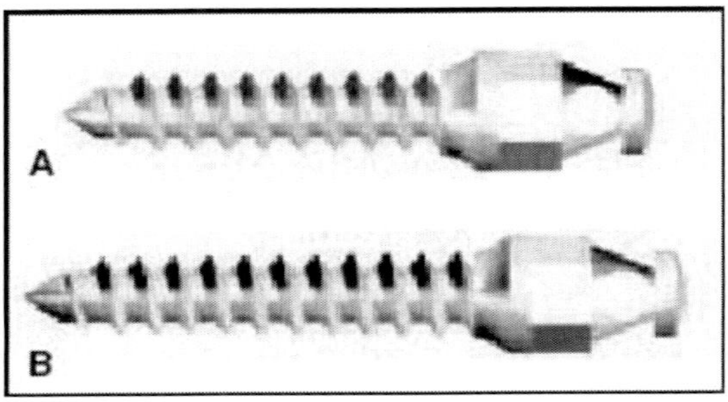

Figure 54. Types of Absoanchor (A) Cylindrical Absoanchor (B) Tapered Absoabchor.

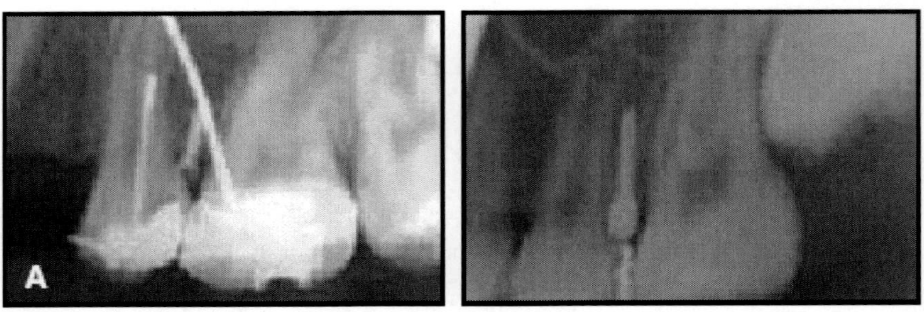

Figure 55. Radiographs after implant placement (A-B) IOPA of second premolar and first molar.

Tapered Absoanchor

The required length of the micro-implant is best judged during pilot drilling. In the mandible, the buccal surfaces and retromolar areas offer adequate thickness and quality of cortical bone for placement of 1.2-1.3mm-diameter micro-implants 4-5mm in length. If lingual micro-implants are needed, the tori are suitable implant sites.

The cortical surfaces of the maxillary buccal area are thinner and less compact than those of the mandible and require longer microimplants generally 6-8mm for a 1.2-1.3mm diameter. The best sites for en masse retraction are the interdental spaces between the second premolars and first molars. Other good maxillary implant sites are below the anterior nasal spine.

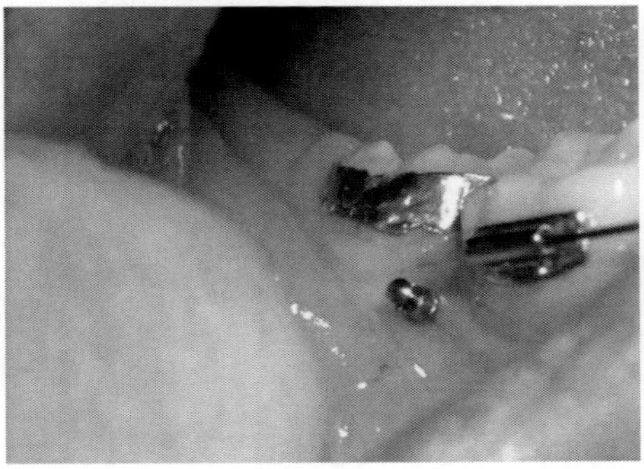

Figure 56. Intraoral Implant placed between first and second molar.

For a palatal implant, the mucosal thickness should be measured with an anesthetic needle or probe. At least 6mm of the microimplant should penetrate into the bone, which usually requires a length of 10-12mm for 1.2-1.3mm-diameter micro-implants placed in the interdental spaces.

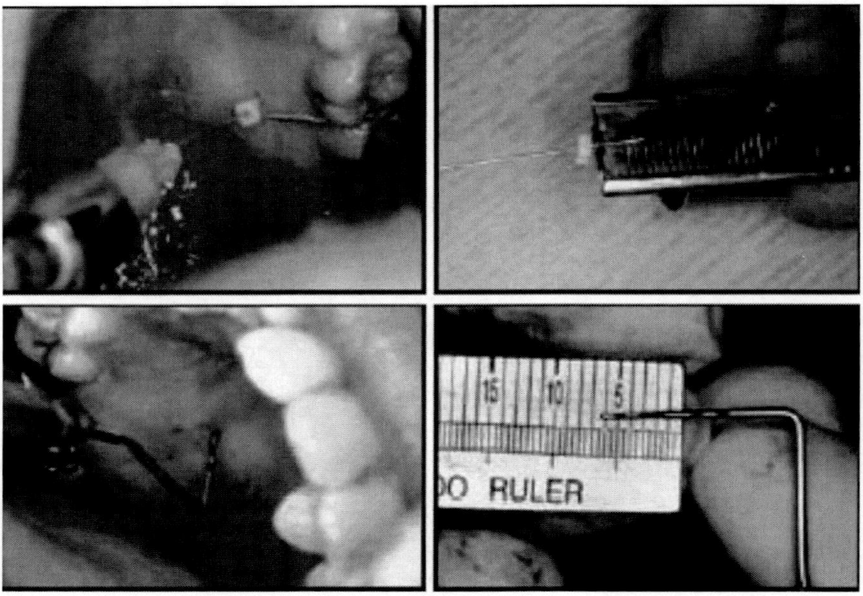

Figure 57. Measurement of soft tissue thickness in Maxillary Arch.

The midline areas contain high-quality cortical bone, but also osseous sutures, so that a micro-implant placed in the suture area should be a little thicker than usual. If the bony resistance of the suture area is inadequate, the micro-implant can be placed adjacent to the suture.

Placement Procedure

A small amount of local anesthetic is sufficient for the simple surgical procedure needed to insert the Absoanchor. The clinician should not try to achieve profound anesthesia of the teeth, but only of the soft tissue. The teeth will be affected only if the bone drill approaches their roots, in which case the drill can be redirected away. When anesthetizing the palatal mucosa, the needle can probe and measure the mucosal thickness and help determine the screw length necessary for anchorage. In extraction cases, Absoanchors can be placed after anesthetizing the teeth for removal, thus avoiding a second surgical procedure.

The implant sites should be marked with brass wires before drilling. Maxillary micro-implant sites need a 30-40° angulation to the long axis of the teeth, either buccally or lingually, to increase the surface contact between the microscrew and the bone.

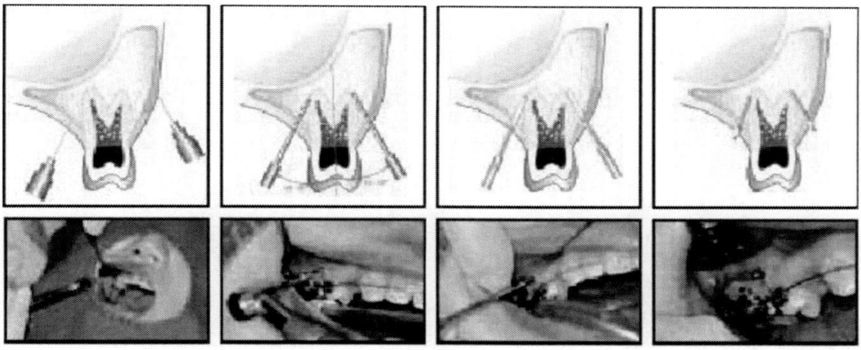

(a) (b) (c) (d)

Figure 58. Placement of Tapered Absoanchor in Maxilla (a) Infiltration anaesthesia before Implant placement (b) Drilling at Implant site (30- 40°) (c) Screwing of Implant with screwdriver (d) Implant placed.

This will improve retention while reducing the risk of striking a root. The thicker mandibular cortical bone generally requires only 10-20° of angulation.

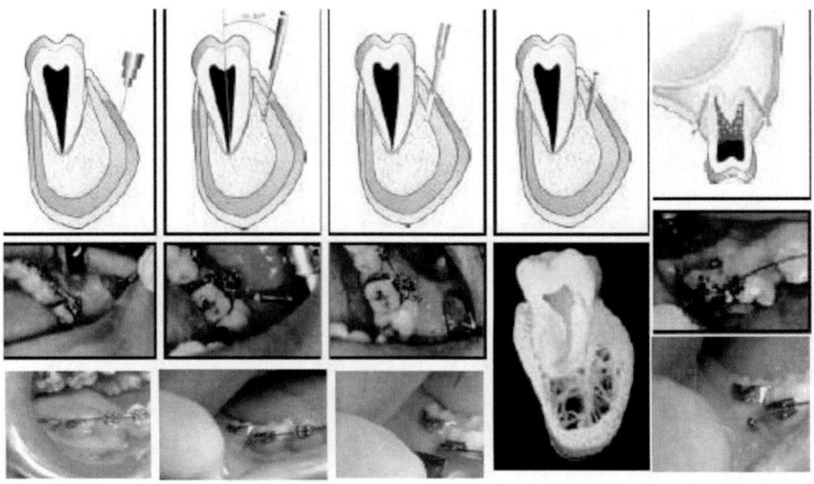

(a) (b) (c) (d) (e)

Figure 59. Placement of Tapered Absoanchor in Mandible (a) Infiltration anaesthesia before Implant placement (b) Drilling at Implant site (10-20°) (c) Screwing of Implant with screwdriver (d) Implant placed.

When placing microimplants in the palate, the greater palatine artery and nerve must always be avoided.

If the micro-implant is inserted through movable soft tissue rather than attached gingiva, it is often preferable to use a screw without a button head, placing it completely beneath the gingiva with an emerging ligature wire hook for elastic attachment. This reduces the risk of inflammation and infection.

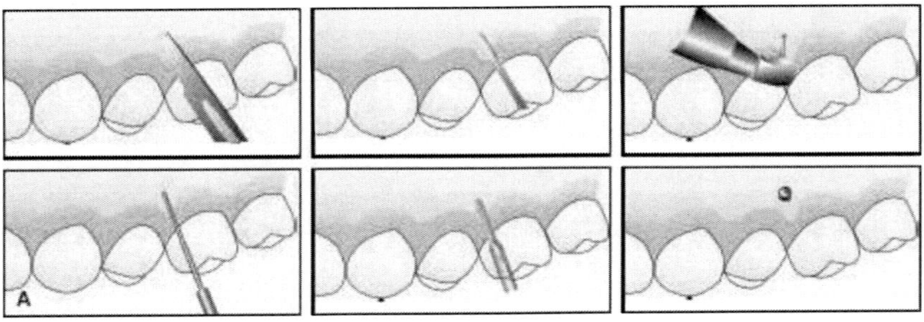

Figure 60. Placement of Tapered Absoanchor in moving soft tissue.

A low-speed contraangle with a drill 0.2-0.3mm narrower than the microscrew is normally used for the initial entry into the bone. The micro-implant itself should not be used for self-drilling, because this can lead to metal fatigue and eventual screw fracture. When using a microscrew narrower than 1.6mm in diameter, the drill should be extended the full length of the screw.

The drill can penetrate the mucosa, attached gingiva, and underlying bone without a surgical flap, but when entering through movable soft tissue, a small (5mm) retractable flap will prevent the soft tissue from rolling up around the drill. A slow drill speed (400-500rpm) should be used with water irrigation to keep the surgical site lubricated. Faster drill speeds of as much as 30,000rpm will work, but run the risk of generating too much heat and thus causing osseous necrosis.

When drilling into dense bone, use careful up-and-down strokes to minimize the heat generated by the low-speed handpiece. Do not use excessive force with the drill. Any serious resistance after passing through the cortical plate is probably due to root contact, which means the drill should be reinserted at a different angle.

An engine-driven screwdriver in a lowspeed contra-angle can be used for placing micro-implants, as in prosthetic dentistry. It is safer to use a manual screwdriver, however, so the clinician can feel any resistance from roots and make adjustments to avoid them. The long screwdriver is designed for buccal surfaces, and the short screwdriver for the palate.

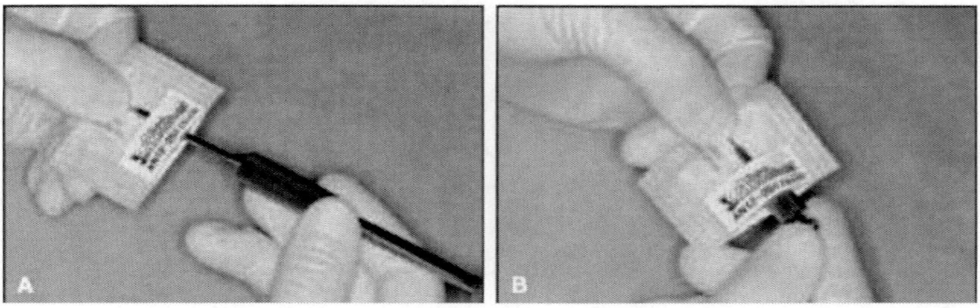

Figure 61. Removal of Absoanchor with screwdriver.

Whenever resistance is encountered, withdraw the implant and redrill the bone with the pilotdrill before reinserting the micro-implant.

If the fit of the micro-implant is not tight enough, replace the implant with the next larger size. Occasionally, a new site adjacent to the original one may need to be prepared. Once the micro-implant fits tightly, orthodontic forces can be applied immediately. Light, continuous forces, as supplied by nickel titanium coil springs, are preferable to the more extreme initial forces of elastomeric modules.

Post-Surgical Management

Excellent home care, including water irrigation, will greatly increase the chances of success. Inflammation due to inadequate oral hygiene can cause even tightly fitting microimplants to loosen. Periodic mouthrinses will help ward off inflammation and infection, and antibiotics can be prescribed as needed. Patients seldom need any medication for pain.

Because complete osseointegration does not occur between the micro-implant and bone, implant removal is simple. Engaging the screw head with the driver and turning it in the opposite direction of insertion will easily remove it without local anesthesia. The patient may experience minor discomfort when the implant contacts the soft tissue, but this is less traumatic than an anesthetic needle-stick.

Transitional Implants

James B. Gray and Robert Smith (2000) [95] used Modular Transitional Implants (MTIs) for orthodontic anchorage. The MTI, 1.8mm in diameter, is available in lengths of 14mm, 17mm and 21mm. It was designed to support a temporary fixed prosthesis during the healing phase associated with placement of permanent implants and to be removed when the permanent implants are restored. The Titanium Modular Transitional Implant is small, affordable, easy to place, routinely resistant to orthodonic forces, able to be immediately loaded, usable with familiar orthodontic mechanics and is easy to remove.

After the vertical dimension had been increased with temporary partial dentures, MTIs were surgically placed under local anesthesia, using a needle-point drill. Pilot-hole channels were drilled in the bone directly through the mucosa to avoid the need for mucoperiosteal flaps. The length of each implant was based on the depth of available bone.

A 21mm MTI was used for indirect orthodontic anchorage distal to the maxillary left first bicuspid, which had been restored with an acrylic crown. An .016 " × .022" nickel titanium wire in a ribbon configuration was bonded with light-cured composite to the slot of the MTI and the occlusal surface of the crown, using a dovetail occlusal preparation. The flexible anchorage of the nickel titanium wire allowed the bicuspid to function occlusally while dissipating these heavier forces at the implant. The bicuspid could then be used to anchor a fixed orthodontic appliance.

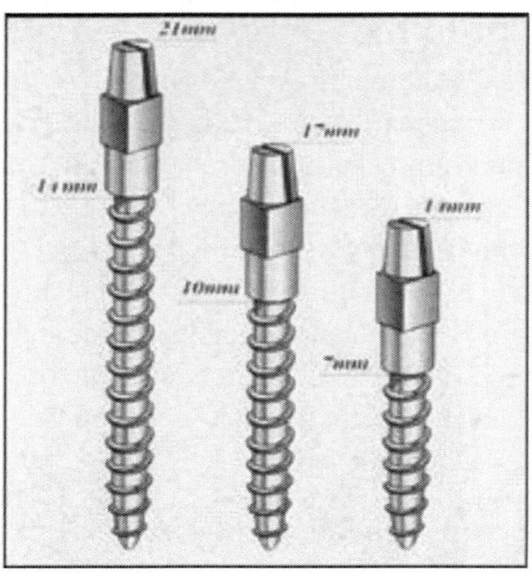

Figure 62. Transitional Implants (21mm, 17mm, 10mm).

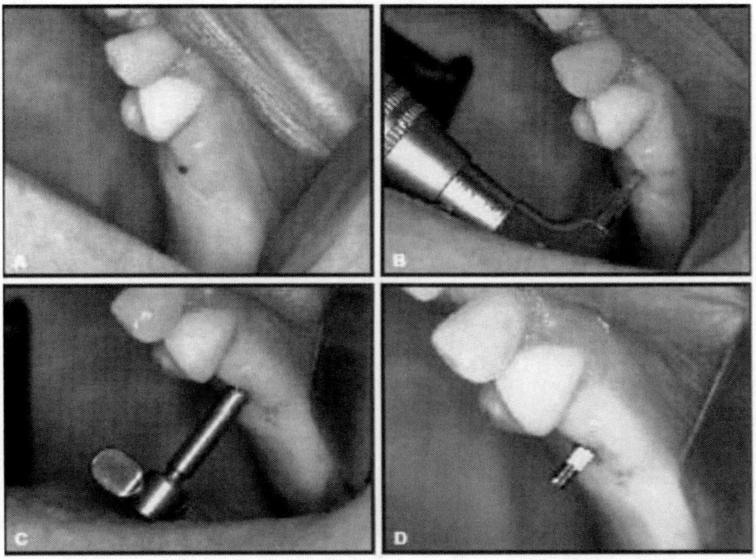

Figure 62. Placement of Transitional Implants. (A) Marking the alveolar gingiva with marker (B) Drilling of the Implant site (C) Implant screwed in with a screwdriver (D) Screwed Implant.

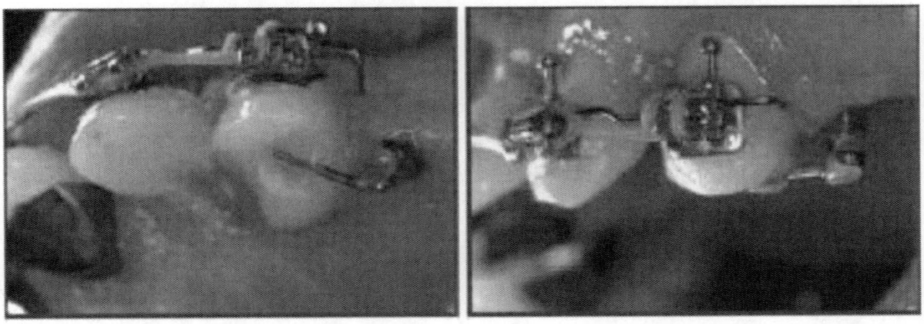

(a) (b)

Figure 63. 0 .016" × .022" nickel titanium wire bonded with light-cured composite to the slot of the MTI and the occlusal surface of the bicuspid crown (a) Occlusal view (b) Buccal view.

Using the available alveolar bone in the maxillary right posterior segment to best advantage, two 17mm MTIs were placed distal to the cuspid (the terminal tooth) for direct orthodontic anchorage.

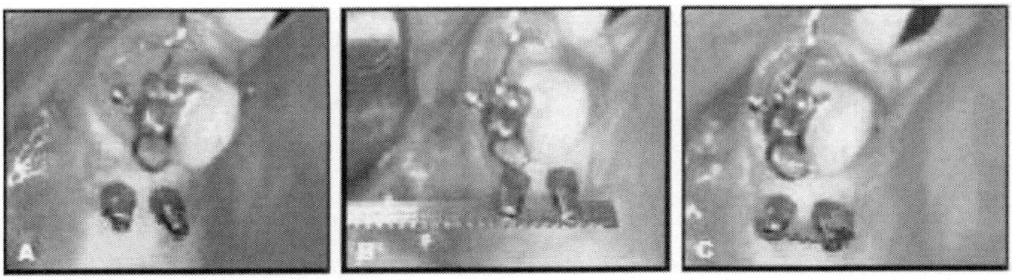

Figure 64. Two 17mm MTIs were placed distal to the cuspid (the terminal tooth) for direct orthodontic anchorage.

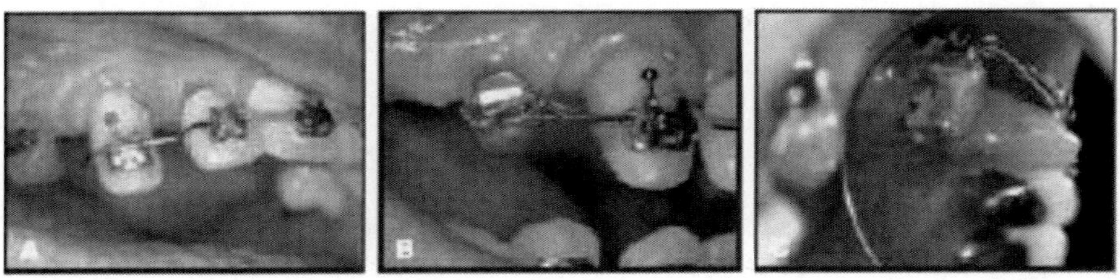

Figure 65. Two 17mm MTIs were placed distal to the cuspid (the terminal tooth) connected with Titanium bar and then covered with light-cure acrylic to simulate a maxillary bicuspid in normal archform.

The MTIs were connected with a titanium bar, which stabilized the implants and prevented their rotation. This apparatus was then covered with light-cure acrylic to simulate a maxillary bicuspid in normal archform. Prior to curing, a mandibular second molar tube with 25° torque was placed upside down in the acrylic.

Aarhus Implant (Birte Melson-1999) [96]

It has a small dimension of 6mm length as a result of which it can be located in multiple sites including between the roots of teeth. It allows osseointegration to occur even in the presence of immediate loading, provided the orthodontic forces (20-50gms) pass through the screw. The strain that develops in the bone surrounding the loaded screw leads to local environment in which increased bone formation results. Due to the size of the screw it can be used in a number of different locations and can be easily removed when no longer required.

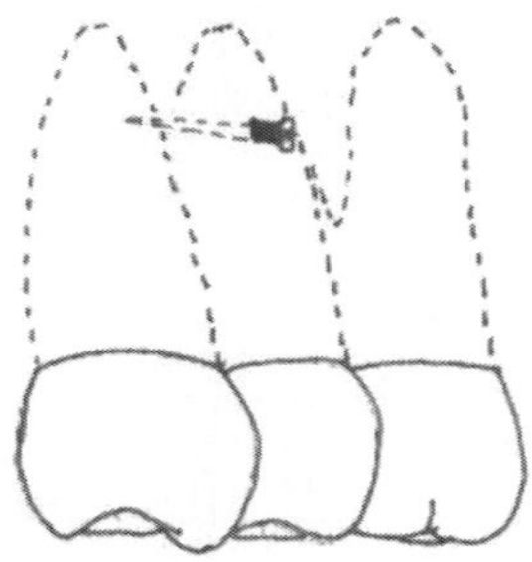

Figure 66. Aarhus Implant.

Graz Implant Supported System (Karcher and Byloff-2000) [97]

Anchorage system consists of a modified titanium miniplate with provision for four miniscrews and two oval shaped cylinders. This was used mainly as a support for the Nance button of a pendulum appliance in the palate.

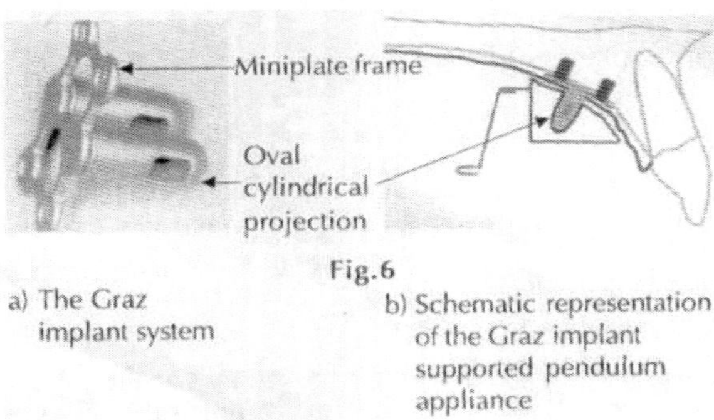

Figure 67. Graz Implant Supported System.

Zygoma Anchor Systems (Clerck and Geerinckx-2002) [98]

It is a curved titanium miniplate with provision of three screws of 2.3mm diameter for stability. The lower end of the miniplate projects outward and contains a vertical slot for ligatures or orthodontic attachments. This system is used in the zygomaticomaxillary buttress area.

Appliance Design and Placement

The upper part of the Zygoma Anchor* is a titanium miniplate with three holes, slightly curved to fit against the inferior edge of the zygomaticomaxillary buttress.

A round bar, 1.5mm in diameter, connects the miniplate and the fixation unit. A cylinder at the end of the bar has a vertical slot, where an auxiliary wire with a maximum size of .032" × .032" can be fixed with a locking screw. The plate is attached above the molar roots by three self-tapping titanium miniscrews, each with a diameter of 2.3mm and a length of 5mm or 7mm. The miniscrews do not need to be sandblasted, etched, or coated. Square holes in the center of the screw heads accommodate a screw-driver for initial placement, while pentagonal outer holes are used to remove the screws at the end of treatment.

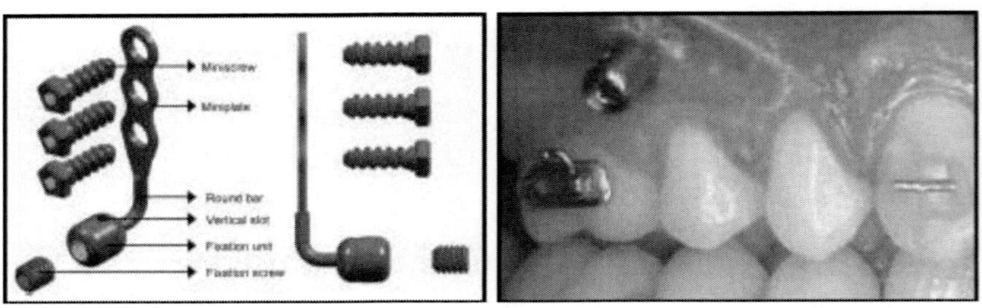

Figure 68. Zygoma Anchor.

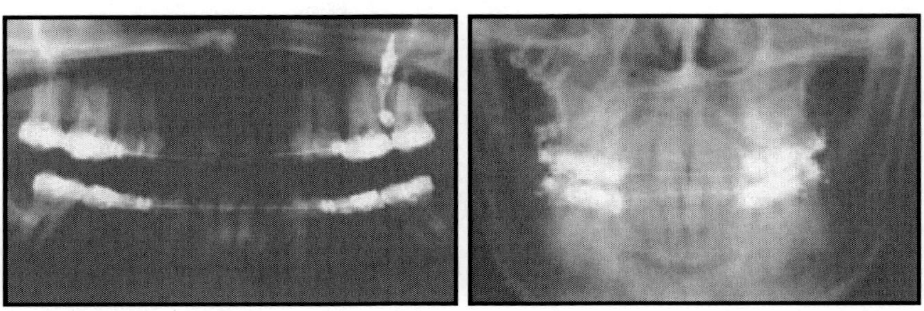

(a) (b)

Figure 69. Zygoma Anchor: Radiographic View (a) OPG (b) Frontal view.

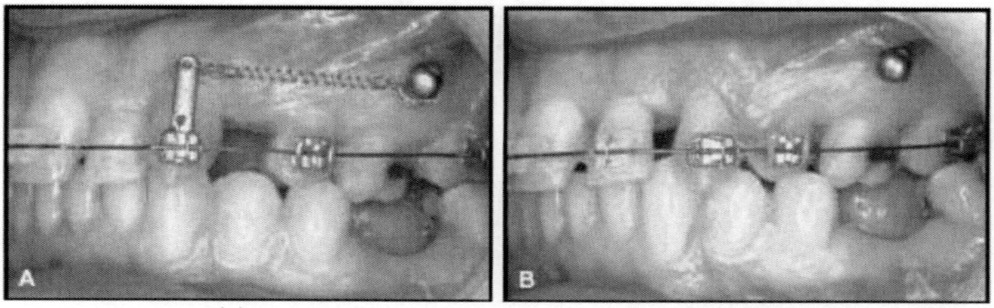

(a) (b)

Figure 70. Zygoma Anchorage System (a) With Rigid Power Arm Attached to Canine (b) After canine distalization.

To place the implant, an L-shaped incision, consisting of a vertical incision mesial to the inferior crest of the zygomaticomaxillary buttress and a small horizontal incision at the border between the mobile and attached gingiva, is made under local anesthesia. The mucoperiosteum is elevated, and the upper part of the anchor is adapted to the curvature of the bone crest. Three holes with a diameter of 1.6mm each are drilled, and the Zygoma Anchor is affixed with the three miniscrews. The cylinder should penetrate the attached gingiva in front of the furcation of the first molar roots at a 90° angle to the alveolar bone surface. When indicated, premolars are extracted at the same appointment.

Biodegradable Implants: (Hashem-2000) [98]

The use of absorbable implants in the repair of bone fractures began in the late 1960's. Fabrication of implants was accomplished by melt moulding and extrusion of polymer into pins and rods.Subsequently more complex designs such as screws and small plates became possible in the late 1970's and early 1980's (Bostman 1991). Alpha compounds such as polyglycolic acid(PGA),poly-l-lactic acid(PLLA) and polyparadioxanon are organic macromolecules that are degradable and absorbable by the body. They also possess the chemical and physical properties necessary for internal fixation devices. The degradation procedure appears to be mainly by hydrolytic activity and to a lesser extent through non-specific enzymatic action. The rate of degradation is dependant on the molecular weight, crystallinity, thermal conductivity, geometry (thin sheet depolymerizes much more rapidly than a dense block of the implant.

The commercially available resorbable polymers include pure polyglycolic (PGA) acid in the form of pins and screws, pure poly-L-lactic acid (PLLA) and a co-polymer of pure PLLA (82%) and PGA (18%) is marketed as LACTOSORB. The features of LACTOSORB include

1. Tensile and flex strength are comparable to titanium plating system.
2. Plates are easy to adapt with aid of heat pack.
3. A wide selection of implant sizes and shapes are available.
4. A convenient hex-drive breakaway delivery system simplifies screw placement.
5. Eliminates growth restriction and implant migration for pediatric craniofacial reconstruction.
6. Resorbs completely and may eliminate the need for second operation.
7. Does not induce late stage inflammatory reaction.

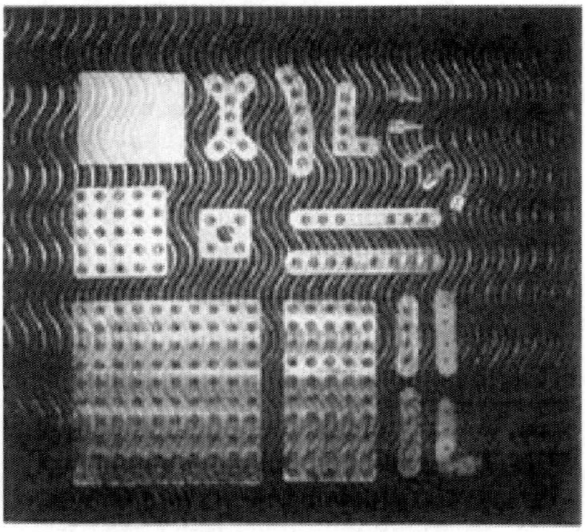

Figure 71. Biodegradable Implants.

C-Microimplant: (Chung-2001) [99]

The C-orthodontic microimplant (Cimplant: Dentium Inc, Seoul, Korea) can be used as an independent orthodontic treatment system in itself as well as an auxiliary to conventional orthodontic mechanics. The 2-component system of the C-implant (screw part and head part) prevents the fracture of the neck area of the fixture during implantation and removal. Also, the long span between head part and screw body prevents gingival irritation during retraction.

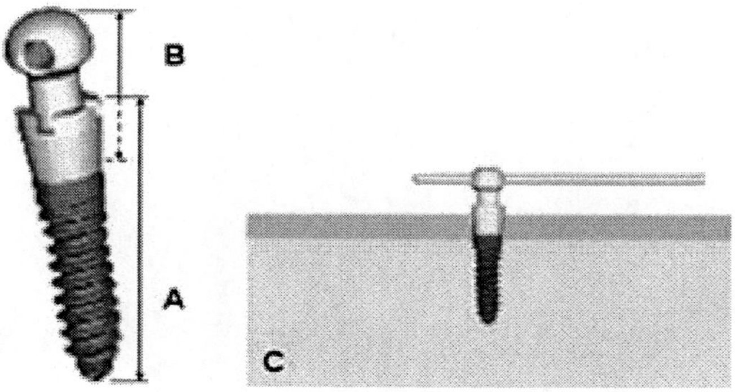

Figure 72. C-orthodontic microimplant (C-implant): (A) screw part (B) head part (C) diagram of placed C-implant.

The screw part has a 1.8-mm diameter and 8.5-, 9.5-, or 10.5-mm length. The surface except for the upper 2 mm is sandblasted, large-grit, and acid etched. The head part has 2.5-mmdiameter and comes in 3 heights: 5.35, 6.35, or 7.35 mm. The distances between the hole of head and screw are 1, 2, or 3 mm, respectively. The diameter of the hole is 0.8 mm.

Implant Placement

After incision of the mucosal area, drilling was carried out at 1500 rpm of drill speed and 15 Ncm of drill pressure with profuse irrigation with isotonic saline solution. The 1.5-mm diameter guide drill (Carl Martin, GmbH, Solingen, Germany) was selected when drilling to depth in cortical bone. The screw part was placed clockwise into the prepared site using internal and external sterile saline cooling. After an 8-week healing period, the head part of C-implant was assembled into the screw part by lightly tapping witha small mallet 1 to 2 times. Immediate loading is possible, mainly in areas where dense bone is located and where primary stability can be achieved.

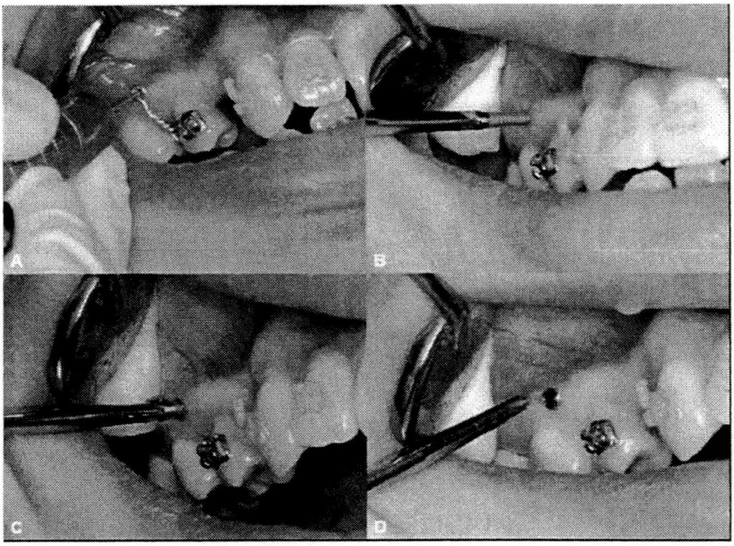

Figure 73. C-implant application procedure (Screw Part). The ligature tie is used to determine the posiition where the implant screw is to be placed. Then the screw is pierced at that point and screwed in with a screwdriver.

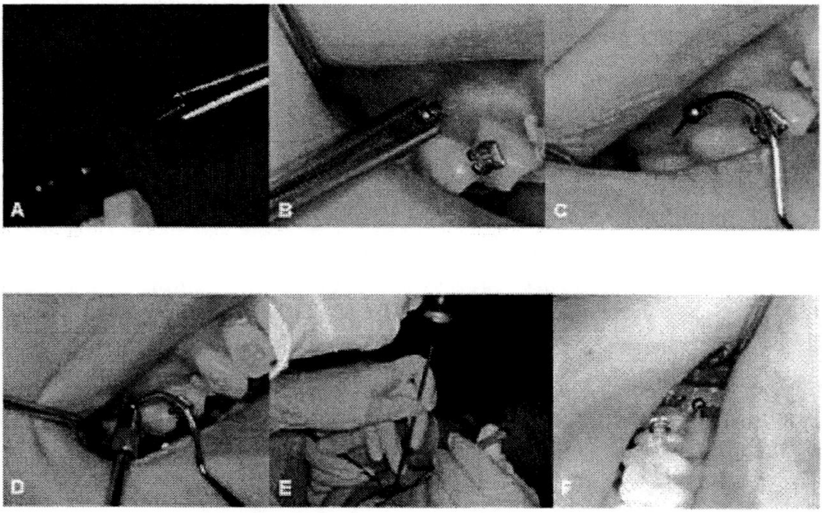

Figure 74. C-implant application procedure (Head Part) (A) C-implant head placed in the beaks of Needle Holder (B) Implant head tightened on screw part (C) Rotation of the head part with explorer (D-E) Tightening of the head part with screwdriver (F) C-implant fully inserted in oral cavity.

Chapter 14

Implants and Distraction Osteogenesis

Mandibular Lengthening Using Osseointegrated Implants

Snyder et al. (1973) [9] published the first report on using distraction osteogenesis to lengthen the canine mandible. Michieli and Miotti (1997) lengthened a dog mandible using an intraoral distraction device attached to the mandibular dentition.

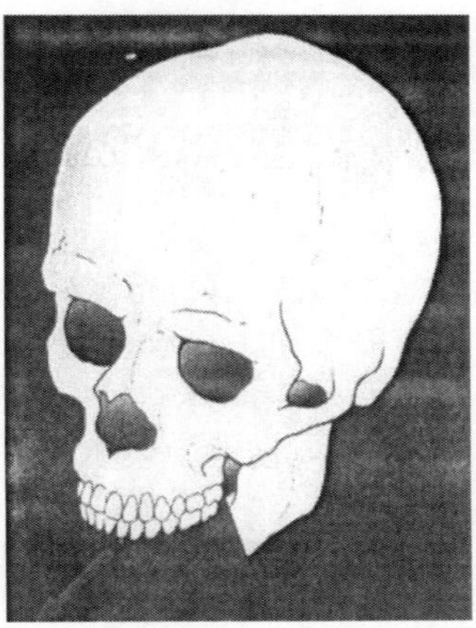

Figure 75. Schematic drawing of mandibular lengthening. Experimental mandibular lengthening in an animal (Sawaki et al. 1996) [9].

Other investigators have also reported successful experimental studies of mandibular lengthening by distraction osteogenesis. In most of these reports, extraoral transcutaneous pins were used to anchor the distraction device. The disadvantages of an extraoral device include extraoral nerve injury and conspicuousness.

Healthy adult male mongrel dogs, each weighing 20 to 25 kg, served as the experimental subjects. The procedure involved five steps: *(1)* tooth extraction, *(2)* implant placement, *(3)* corticotomy and device setting, *(4)* distraction, and *(5)* fixation.

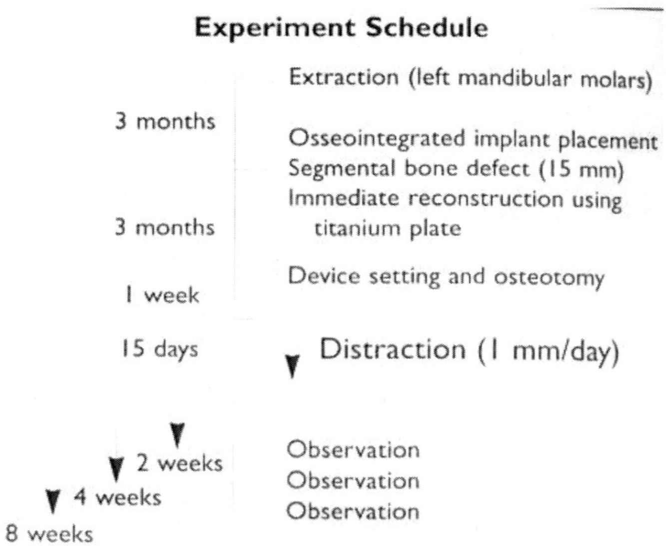

Figure 76. Experiment schedule of mandibular lengthening.

The left mandibular pre-molars were extracted 2 months before implant placement. Two endosseous titanium implants were placed 30 mm apart in the left mandible of each dog. The implants were cylindrical, threaded, 10 mm long, and 3.75 mm in diameter. The relationship of the implants to each other was transferred by implant mounts and stainless bars; acrylic resin was used for making the superstructure.

The implants were surgically exposed after 3 months. Standard abutments, 5.5 mm in length, were connected to the osseointegrated implants with abutment screws. After the device was adjusted, a subperiosteal corticotomy around the mandible using a fissure bur in an electrical handpiece created an artificial fracture between the implants to give mobility to the segments.

Finally, the distraction device was connected to abutments so that the proximal and distal bone fragments could be fixed. After a 10-day healing of the periosteum, the distraction was performed at the rate of 1 mm per day, in accordance with Ilizarov, for 10 consecutive days to elongate the bone by 10 mm. Then the device was stabilized with acrylic resin.

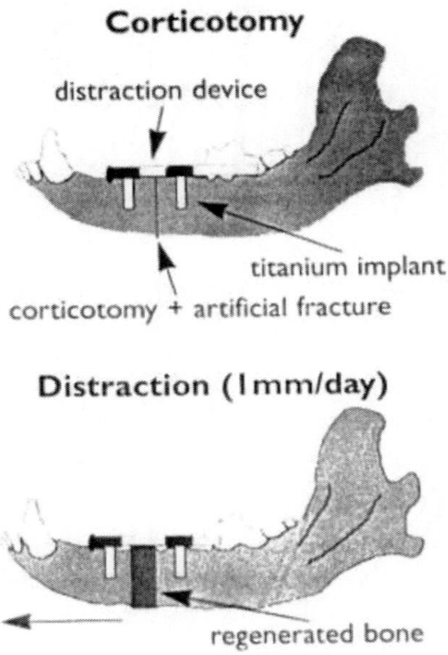

Figure 77. Procedure of distraction – corticotomy followed by formation of regenerated bone.

Radiographs were obtained before and after corti-cotomy, immediately before initial distraction, at days 5 and 10 during distraction, and at 1 week intervals after completion of distraction.

At 2, 4, 6, and 8 weeks animals were sacrificed.

Bone Healing of Mandible after Distraction

During the experimental period, there were no problems with the host or the device. All the animals tolerated the operation and distraction well. Furthermore, the distraction device remained stable.

Morphological findings demonstrated definite elongation of the mandible, a resulting shift of the mandible to the right, and a severe crossbite.

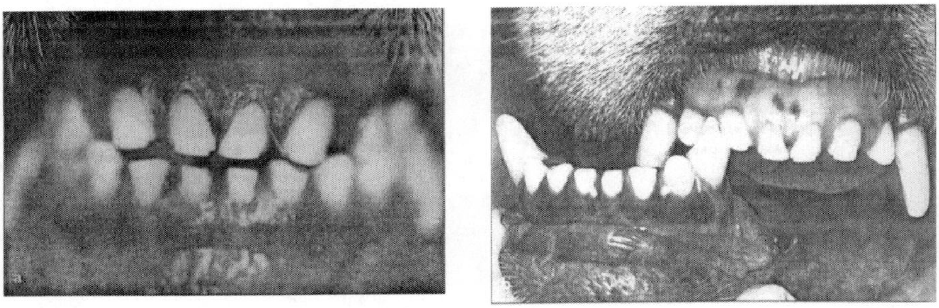

(a) (b)

Figure 78. (a) Before distraction in dog mandible (b) After distraction a resulting shift of the mandible to the right and a severe crossbite developed.

The distance between the two abutments was found to be 10 mm greater than preoperatively. The soft tissues were intact and normal in appearance. The gingiva around the abutments and wounds from incision and suturing showed normal healing. None of the implants had lost osseo-integration. Bimanual palpation showed that the elongated site had elastic hardness and mobility 2 weeks after completion of distraction and gradually became firm by 6 weeks. No abnormal healing of fracture, such as fibrous union or pseudoarthrosis, was found in any cases.

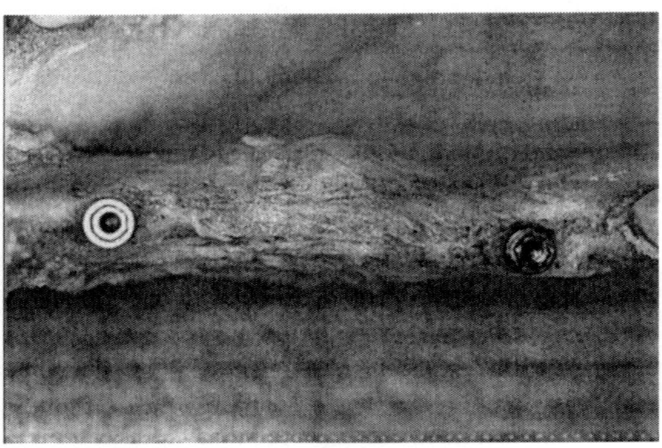

Figure 79. Increased distance between the abutments after distraction.

The axial radiograph of the mandible initially showed a line of radiolucency corresponding to the corticotomy. The width of the line began to decrease during the waiting period, indicating the start of bone healing. As distraction began, the mandible was separated into proximal and distal segments. At the end of distraction, the lengthened area was found to be a clear radiolucent space. In the occlusal radiograph, the edges of the distraction gap were clearly observed 2 weeks after the completion of distraction, and parallel columns of bone extended from the cut edges toward a central radiolucent zone. By 4 weeks, bone was found bridging the gap, with the radiolucent zone diminishing. By 6 and 8 weeks, radiopacity of the gap became more advanced, indicating further maturation. Moreover, no bone resorption was observed around the titanium implants.

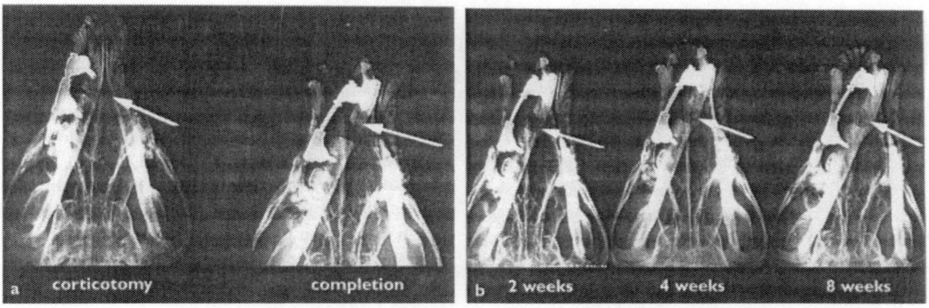

Figure 80. Axial radiograph showing lengthening of mandible with Increase in radio-opaque area at 2, 4 and 8 weeks.

Histological sections showed connective tissue in the distraction gap 2 weeks after completion of distraction. Collagen fibers were rectilinear, stretched out, and oriented in the tension vector. The short, immature (woven) bone, oriented in the direction of the distraction, was shown to be close to the proximal edges of the corticotomy. At 4 weeks, regenerated bone close to the edges demonstrated more advanced calcification, and networks of immature bone were formed. The central radiolucent zone was composed of the woven bone and connective tissue. This finding seemed to reflect the characteristic structure shown radiographically. At 6 weeks, the distraction gap was filled with a network of newly formed bone. However, various stages of bone maturation and two types of ossification could be seen within the same specimen. The main histological feature was fairly mature bone that had a lamellar structure surrounding vascular canals. On the surface of the new bone, the arrangement of active osteoblasts was visible on a layer of lighter-stained primary bone. There were also some fibrocartilage islands in the central radi-olucent area and near the proximal end. New bone had been formed in the matrix of hypertrophic chondrocytes. At 8 weeks, regenerated bone close to the proximal segments had acquired a mature lamellar structure.

Maxillary Advancement Using Osseointegrated Implants

Advancement of the anterior maxilla is often required to correct skeletal deformity and malocclu-sion. Block and Brister (1994) showed the possibility of maxillary advancement in the dog by distraction osteogenesis, using an intraoral device supported by the teeth.

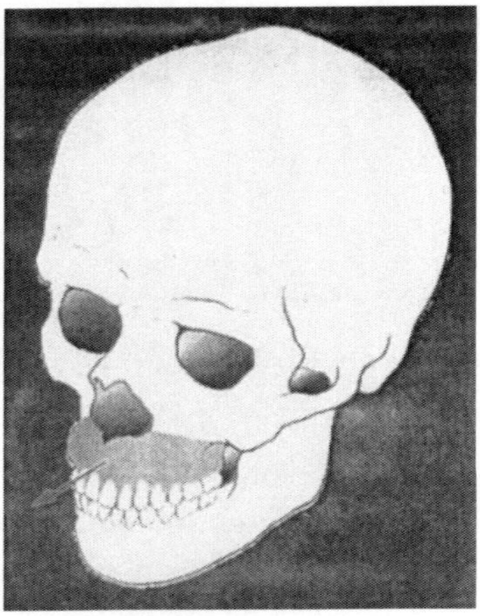

Figure 81. Experimental maxillary advancement in an animal (Yamamoto et al. 1997) [9].

According to the experiment schedule, premolars and molars were extracted from the maxilla and, after 3 months, four osseoin-tegrated titanium implants were placed in the alveolar ridge. The implants were cylindrical, threaded, 10 mm long, and 3.75 mm in diameter.

After 3 months, abutments (5.5 mm in length) were connected to the implants and the osteotomy was performed. Vestibular incisions were made to expose the lateral maxillary walls and the piriform rim, and the mucosa was elevated to expose the bony nasal floor. Osteotomy was performed from the lateral maxilla to the piriform rim using a reciprocating saw and a fissure bur. The medial portion of the implants in the palate was separated in the same manner. When the osteotomy had been completed, the anterior bone segment could be mobilized manually. The mucosal incision was closed with 5-0 nylon sutures. Finally, the originally fabricated distraction device, consisting of an orthodontic rapid expansion screw, was connected to the abutments.

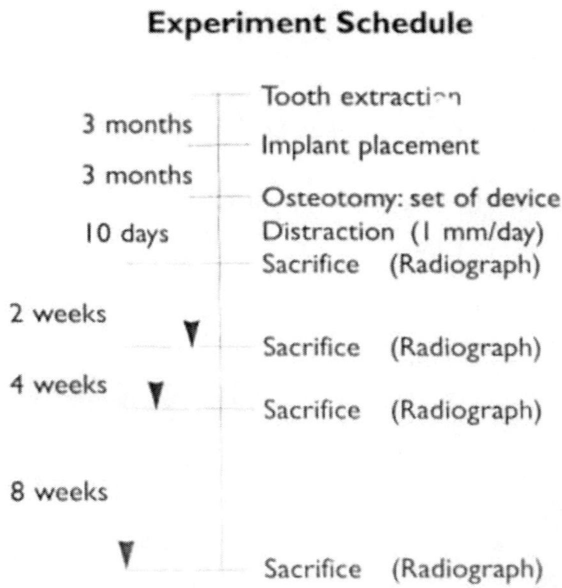

Figure 82. Experimental Schedule for maxillary advancement.

Ten days after the operation, distraction was performed at the rate of 1 mm per day for 10 consecutive days. After achieving elongation of 10 mm, the device was used to stabilize the bone segments.

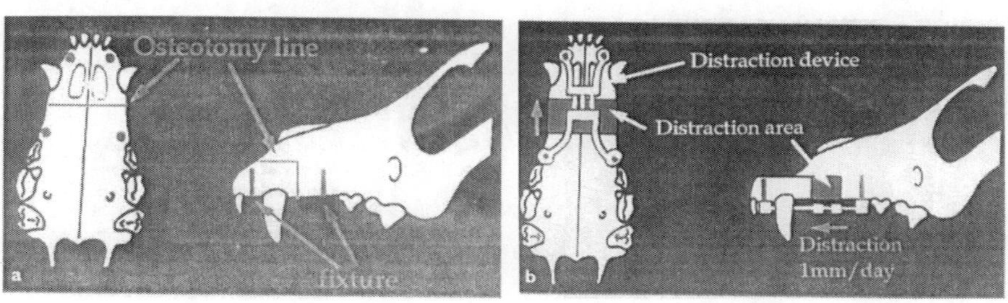

Figure 83. Maxillary advancement (a) Osteotomy line (b) Distraction area.

At 2, 4, and 8 weeks after fixation, morphological and radiographic observations were carried out simultaneously and the specimens, including the distraction gap, were harvested for histological examination. Each maxillary bone was removed, and each specimen was prepared in the usual manner and stained with hematoxylin-eosin. Tissues surrounding the implant were then observed under nondecalcified staining with toluidine blue stain.

Bone Healing of Maxilla after Distraction

Morphological observations after distraction showed a definite anterior protrusion of the maxilla with no adverse soft tissue reaction 8 weeks after fixation. From the occlusal view, a definitive elongation of the premaxilla and a severe overjet were observed.

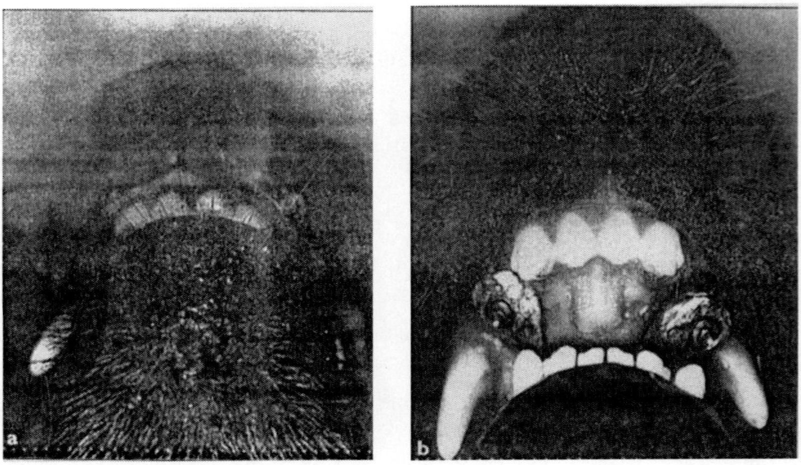

(a) (b)

Figure 84. Maxillary advancement occlusal view (a) Before advancement (b) After advancement.

Upon gross examination of the removed maxilla, the distracted area was found to be filled with newly formed bone; fibrous tissue became indistinguishable as the stabilization period lengthened. Eight weeks after fixation, the matured bone that had formed in the distraction gap became hard to the touch.

Radiological observations showed a typical healing process. The farther the anterior maxillary segment advanced during distraction, the wider the radiolucent area created at the osteotomy site became. Calcification in the distraction gap increased so as to become symmetrical and uniform. After 2 weeks of fixation, the distraction gap showed rounding of the bony edges, and after 4 weeks new bone was found bridging the gap; by 8 weeks the border between original and regenerated bone was difficult to distinguish. Soft-ray radiographs of the removed maxillary specimen showed that as the stabilization period became longer more and more radiopaque bone filled the distracted area. All the anterior bone segments had advanced; the radiographs revealed increased radiodensity of the bone, making it indistinguishable from the original bony edges as the area filled with mature bone tissue.

Histological findings showed that the gap had filled with fibrous connective tissue within 2 weeks. The course of the fibers was in the same direction the bone was pulled. The development of newly formed bone, indicating lamellar structures along the fiber bundles from one part of the bone stump, was evident. Osteoblasts, osteoids, and pre- calcification of newly formed bone were seen on the side of the marrow cavity, indicating the presence of active osteogenesis.

During the fourth week after fixation, active outgrowth of newly formed bone was observed along the fiber length, developing toward the center portion. In the sixth week, the bone gap had completely filled with mature bone and was continuous with the matrix bone. Observation of the implant-bone interface 6 weeks after fixation showed no fibrous connective tissue around the implant, which was surrounded by mature, newly formed bone having no inflammatory cellular infiltration.

Conclusion

Osseointegrated implants for the purpose of conserving anchorage are welcome additions to the armamentarium of a clinical orthodontist. Implants are now being used to enhance more traditional orthodontic techniques. In particular, they have the potential to provide a useful method of anchorage reinforcement, particularly in cases otherwise dependant on patient compliance. The continuing development of orthodontic implants has led to the production of smaller designs which are easy to insert and remove, and do not require a long healing period prior to loading. They help the orthodontist to overcome the challenge of unwanted reciprocal tooth movement.

In the future, as developments occur in implant technology, they have significant role as anchorage reinforcement aids in place of headgears. However, the presently available implant systems are bound to change into more patient friendly and operator convenient designs.

Bibliography

[1] Linkow L I. 1968. "The blade-vent-a new dimension in endosseous implants." *Dent Conc.* 3:11.

[2] Kenneth J A. 1996. *Phillip's Science of Dental Materials.* 10th edition, W.B Saunders company.

[3] Driskell T D. 1987. "History of implants." *J. Calif. Dent. Assoc.* 15:17.

[4] Harris S M. 1887. "An artificial tooth." Quoted in *Dent. Cosmos.* 55:433.

[5] Bonwell. 1913. "First District Dental Society: In Greenfield EG: Implantation of Artificial Bridge Abutments." *Dent. Cosmos* 55:364.

[6] Payne R E. 1901. "Implantation of teeth by silver capsule." *Dent. Cosmos. 12*:14.

[7] Greenfield E J. 1913. "Implantation of artificial crown and bridge abutments." *Dent. Cosmos.* 55:364.

[8] Adams P B. "Anchoring means for false teeth." U. S Patent No. 2, 112,007, March 22, 1938.

[9] Block M S, Kent J N, Guerra L R. 2000. *Implants in Dentistry*; Ist Edition, W.B Saunders Company.

[10] Branemark P I. "Introduction to Osseointegration." *In Branemark P I* et al. *(eds) Tissue Integrated Prostheses.* Chicago, Quintessence Publishing Co, In.

[11] Gainsforth B L, Higley L B. 1945. "A study of orthodontic anchorage possibilities in basal bone." *Am. J. Orthod. Oral. Surg.* 31: 406-17.

[12] Sherman A J.1978. "Bone reaction to orthodontic forces on vitreous carbon dental implants." *Am. J. Orthod.* 74: 79-87.

[13] Smith J R.1979. "Bone dynamics associated with the controlled loading of bioglass-coated aluminum endosteal implants." *Am. J. Orthod.* 76:618-36.

[14] Guyman G W, Kokich V G, and Oswald R J. 1980. "Ankylosed teeth as abutments for palatal expansion in the rhesus monkey." *Am. J. Orthod.* 77: 486-99.

[15] Gray J B, Steen M E, King G J, Clark A E.1983. "Studies of the efficacy of implants as orthodontic anchorage." *Am. J. Orthod.* 83: 311-317.

[16] Roberts W E, Smith R K, Zilberman Y, Mozsary P G.1984. "Osseous adaptation to continuous loading of rigid endosseous implants." *Am. J. Orthod.* 86:95-111.

[17] Smalley W M, Shapiro P A, Hohl T H, Kokich V G, Brånemark P-I.1988. "Osseointegrated titanium implants for maxillofacial protraction in monkeys." *Am. J. Orthod. Dentofacial Orthop.* 94:285-95.

[18] Turley, P K et al.1989. "Orthodontic force application to titanium endosseous implants." *Angle Orthod.* 58:151-162.

[19] Roberts W E, Helm R R, Marshall K J, Gongloff R K.1989. "Rigid endosseous implants for orthodontic and orthopedic anchorage." *Angle Orthod.* 59: 247-256.

[20] Roberts, W E. Marshall, K J and Mozsary P G.1990."Rigid endosseous implant utilized as anchorage to protract molars and close an atrophic extraction site." *Angle Orthod.* 60:135-152.

[21] Block M S, Hoffman D R.1995."A new device for absolute anchorage for orthodontics." *Am. J. Orthod. Dentofacial Orthop.* 107:251-258.

[22] Southard T E, Buckley M J, Spivey J D, Krizan K E, Casko J S.1995."Intrusion anchorage potential of teeth versus rigid endossseous implants: a clinical and radiographic evaluation." *Am. J. Orthod. Dentofacial Orthop.* 107:115-20.

[23] Parr J A, Garetto L P, Wohlford M E, Arbuckle G R, Roberts W E. 1997." Sutural expansion using rigidly integrated endosseous implants: An experimental study in rabbits." *Angle Orthod.* 4:283-90.

[24] Akin-Nergiz N, Nergiz A, Arpak N, Schulz A, Neidermeier W. 1998."Reactions of peri-implant tissues to continuous loading of osseointegrated implants." *Am. J. Orthod. Dentofacial Orthop.* 114:292-98.

[25] De Pauw G A M, Dermaut L, De Bruyn H, Johanssen C.1999. "Stability of implants as anchorage for orthopedic traction." *Angle Orthod.* 69:401-407.

[26] Weihrbein H, Merz B R, Deidrich P.1999."Palatal bone support for orthodontic implant anchorage—a clinical and radiologic study." *Eur. J. Orthod.* 21:65-70.

[27] Majzoub Z, Finotti M, Miotti F, Giardino R, Aldini N N, Cordioli G. 1999. "Bone response to orthodontic loading of endosseous implants in the rabbit calvaria: early continous distalisation." *Eur. J. Orthod.* 21:223-30.

[28] Saito S, Sugimoto N, Morohashi T, Ozeki M, Kurabayashi H, Shimizu H, Yamasaki K, Shiba A, Yamada S, Shibasaki Y.2000. "Endosseous titanium implants as anchors for mesiodistal Tooth movement in the beagle dog." *Am. J. Orthod. Dentofacial Orthop.* 122:566-70.

[29] Daimaruya T, Nagasaka H, Umemori M, Sugawara J, Mitani H.2001."The influence of molar intrusion on the inferior alveolar neurovascular bundle and root using the skeletal anchorage system in dogs." *Angle Orthod.* 71:60-70.

[30] Ohmae M, Saito S, Morohashi T,Seki K,Qu H,Kanomi R.2001. "A clinical and histological evaluation of titanium mini-implants as anchors for orthodontic intrusion in the beagle dog." *Am. J. Orthod. Dentofacial Orthop.* 119;489-97.

[31] Thilander B,Odman J, Lekholm U.2001."Orthodontic aspects of the use of oral implants in adolescents:a 10 year follow-up study."*Eur. J. Orthod.* 23:715-31.

[32] Gedrange T, Bourauel C, Kobel C, Harzer W.2003. "Three dimensional analysis of endosseous palatal implants and bones after vertical, horizontal,and diagonal force application." *Eur. J. Orthod.* 25:109-115.

[33] Erverdi N, Keles A, Nanda R.2004."The use of skeletal anchorage in open bite treatment: A cephalometric evaluation." *Angle Orthod.* 74:381-90.

[34] Aldikacti M, Acikgoz G, Turk T, Trisi P. 2004."Long-term evaluation of sandblasted and acid etched implants used as orthodontic anchors in dogs." *Am. J. Orthod. Dentofacial Orthop.* 125:139-147.

[35] Sugawara J, Daimaruya T, Umemori M, Nagasaki H, Takahashi I, Kawamura H, Mitani H. 2004."Distal movement of mandibular molars in adult patients with the skeletal anchorage system." *Am. J. Orthod. Dentofacial Orthop.* 125:130-138.

[36] Oyonarte R, Pilliar R M, Woodside D.2005. "Peri-implant bone response to orthodontic loading:Part I. A histomorphometric study of the effects of implant surface design." *Am. J. Orthod. Dentofacial Orthop.* 128:173-181.

[37] Lemons J, Natiella J. 1986."Biomaterials, biocompatibility and peri-implant considerations." *Dent. Clin. North Am.* 30:4.

[38] Goldberg M I, Gershkoff A.1949. "The implant lower denture." *Dent. Dig.* 55:490.

[39] Cranin A N, et al. 1987. "Evolution of dental implant in the twentieth century." *Alpha Omegan* 80:25.

[40] Berman N.1952. "The physiologist and mechanical aspect of the implant technique and its application to practical cases." *Dent. Dig.* 8:342.

[41] Bodine R L.1963."Implant dentures: Follow-up after 7-10 years." *J. Am. Dent. Assoc.* 67:352-363.

[42] Izikowitz L. 1962. "Superplants." *J. Implant Dent.* 8:18-32.

[43] Lee T C.1970. "History of dental implants." In Cranin AN (ed) *Oral implantology. Springfield, Ill*, Charles C Thomas pp 3-5.

[44] Lew I.1959. "Progress in implant dentistry: An evalution." *J. Am. Dent. Assoc.* 59:478-92.

[45] Weinberg L.1970. "An early unilateral subperiosteal implant." In Cranin AN (ed) *Oral Implantology. Springfield, Ill,* Charles C Thomas, p 19.

[46] Golec TS.1986. "CAD CAM multiplanar diagnostic imaging for subperiosteal implants." *Dent. Clin. North Am.* 30:85.

[47] Babbush C A. 1989. *personal communication.*

[48] Small I A.1978. "Metal implants and the mandibular staple bone plate." *Oral. Surg.* 36:604.

[49] Small I A. 1975. "Metal implants and the mandibular staple bone plate." *Oral. Surg.* 33:571.

[50] Small I A, Misiek D J. 1984. "A 16 year evalution of the mandibular staple bone plate." *J. Oral. Maxillofac. Surg.* 42:421-28.

[51] Cranin AN, Dennison T.1970. "The anterior vertical transosseous implant." In Cranin AH (ed) *Oral Implantology. Springfield Ill*, Carles C Thomas, pp 200-08.

[52] Bosker H, Van Dijk L.1989. "The transmandibular implants: A 12-year follow –up study." *J. Oral. Maxillofac. Surg.* 147:442-450.

[53] Proceeding of the toronto conferences on Osseointegration in Clinical Dentistry.1993. *J. Prosth Dent.* 49:50.

[54] Branemark P I. 1985. "Introduction to Osseointegration." *In Branemark PI* et al. *(eds) Tissue Integrated Prostheses.* Chicago, Quintessence Publishing Co, In p 29.

[55] Adell R, Lekholm U, Rocker B, Branemark PI.1981. "A 15 year study of osseontegrated implants in the treatment of the edentulous jaw." *Int. J. Oral. Surg.* 10:387.

[56] Zarb G.1991."Implants for complete denture therapy." *J. Dent. Educ.* 152:721.

[57] Curriculum Guidelines for predoctoral implant dentistry.1991. *J. Dent. Educ.* 55:751-53.

[58] English C.1990. "An overview of implant hardware." *J. Am. Dent. Assoc.* 121:360-70.

[59] Driskell T D, O'Hara M J, Greene G W.1971. "Surgical tooth implants, combat and field." Report No. 1, Contract No. DA DA17-69-c-9118. Supported by U.S. Army Medical Research an Development Command.

[60] Kirsh A, Mentag P.1986. "The IMZ endosseous two-phase system: A complete oral rehabilitation treatment concept." *J. Oral. Impl.* 12.

[61] Schroedar A et al.1976. "Tissue reaction to a titanium hollow cylinder implant with titanium plasma spread layer surface." *Schweiz Mschr Zahnleilk* 86:713.

[62] Suter F, et al.1983. "ITI hollow cylinder system: Principles and methodology." *J. Oral. Implantology* 11:168.

[63] Niznick G A. 1982. "The Core-Vent Implant system." *Oral Implantol.* 10:379-418.

[64] Kent J et al.1990. "Biointegrated hydroxylapatite coated dental implants: Five year clinical observation." *Jam Dent. Assoc.* 121:138-144.

[65] Linkow L I.1969. "The endosseous blade implant and its use in orthodontics." *Int. J. Orthod.* 18:149-54.

[66] Shulman L B.1985. "Dental replantation and transplantation." In Louis, CV Mosby, pp 132, 133, 136.

[67] Dahl G S A.1943. "Om impjlighenten for implantation I Keken au meteliskelett som has eller retention for fastoc eller avatagbara protesor." (Mandibular subperiosteal implants.) *Odontol. Tidskr* 51:440.

[68] Marziani L.1947. "Redici artificidi come ancoraggio de protesi complete mobile interior." *Clin. Odont.* 2:224.

[69] Linkow L I.1968. "The blade-vent – a new dimension in endosseous implants." *Dent Cong.* 11:3.

[70] Robert H D, Robert R A.1970." The ramus endosseous implant." *J. South Calif. Dent. Assoc.* 38:571.

[71] Zarb G.1983. Proceeding. Toronto conference on Osseointegration in Clinical Dentistry. St. Louis, CV Mosby.

[72] Kasemo B.1983. "Biocompatibility of Titanium Implants: Surface science aspects." *J. Prosth* 49:832-837.

[73] Adell R, Lekholm U, Rocker B, And Branemark P I.1981." A 15-year study of osseointegrated implants in the treatment of the endosseous jaw." *Int. J. Oral. Surg.* 6:387.

[74] Higuchi K W, Branemark P I.2000. *Osseointegrated Implants;Ist Edition*,Quintessence Publishing Company.

[75] Tencate A R.1985. "The gingival junction." In Branemark P-I, Zarb G A, Albrektsson T (eds) *Tissue Integrated Prostheses-Osseointegration in Clinical Dentistry*. London, Quintessence Publishing Co.Inc.,pp 145-153.

[76] Albrektsson T, Branemark P I, Hansson H A, Kasemo B, Larsson K, Lundstrom I, McQueen D H, Skalak R.1983. "The interface Zone of inorganic implants in vivo: Titanium implants in bone." *Ann. Biomed. Eng.* 11:1–27.

[77] Carlsson L et al.1988. "Implant fixation improved by close fit."*Acta Orthop. Scand.* 59:272-75.

[78] Soballe K et al.1990. "Hydroxyapatite coating enhances fixation of porous coated implants." *Acta Orthop. Scand.* 61:299-306.

[79] Movassaghi et al.1995. "Frontonasal suture expansion in rabbits using titanium screws."*J. Oral. Max Surg.*

[80] Kokich V G, Shapiro P A, Oswald R, Koskinen-Moffett L, Clarren S K. 1985. "Ankylosed teeth as abutments for maxillary protraction." *Am. J. Orthod. Dentofacial Orthop.* 88:303-07.

[81] Roberts W E, Nelson C L, Goodacre C J.1994. "Rigid Implant Anchorage to Close a Mandibular First Molar Extraction Site." *Am. J. Othod. Dentofacial Orthop.* Dec:693-704.

[82] Umemori M, Sugawara J, Mitani H, Nagasaka H, and Kawamura H.1999. "Skeletal anchorage system for open-bite correction." *Am. J. Orthod.* 115:166-174.

[83] Creekmore T D and Eklund M K.1983. "The possibility of skeletal anchorage." *J. Clin. Orthod.* 17:266-269.

[84] Bousquet F, Bousquet P, Mauran G,Parguel P.1996. "Use of an impacted post for anchorage." *J. Clin. Orthod.* 30:261-65.

[85] Isono H, Kaida K, Hamada Y, Kokubo Y, Ishihara M, Hirashita A, Kuwahara Y.2002. "The reconstruction of bilateral clefts using endosseous implants after bone grafting." *Am. J. Orthod. Dentofacial Orthop* 121:403-10.

[86] Kanomi R.1997. "Mini-implant for orthodontic anchorage." *J. Clin. Orthod.* 31:763-67.

[87] Celenza F, Hochman M N.2000. "Absolute anchorage in orthodontics: Direct and indirect implant-assisted modalities." *J. Clin. Orthod.* 34:397-402.

[88] Park H, Bae S, Kyung H, Sung J, Kim I.2003. "Development of Intra-oral Micro-Implants for Orthodontic Anchorage." *J. Clin. Orthod.* 37:321-32.

[89] Gray J B, Smith R.2000. "Transitional implants for orthodontic anchorage." *J. Clin. Orthod.* 34:659-66.

[90] Ismail S F H, Johal A S.2002."The role of implants in orthodontics." *Jour. Orthod.* 29:239-245.

[91] Byloff F K, Karcher H, Clar E, Stoff F.2000. "An implant to eliminate abchorage loss during molar distalization: a case report involving the Graz implant-supported pendulum." *Int. J. Adult Orthon. Orthognath Surg.* 15:129-37.

[92] De Clerk H, Geerinckx V, Siciliano S.2002."The Zygoma Anchorage System." *Jour. Clin. Orthod.* 36:455-459.

[93] Mohammed-Hashem I K, Mitchell D A.2000. "Resorbable implants in orthognathic surgery."*Jour. Orthod.* 27:198-199.

[94] Chung K, Kim S, Kook Y. 2004. "C-Orthodontic Microimplant for Distalization of Mandibular Dentition in Class II Correction Resorbable implants in orthognathic surgery." *Angle Orthod.* 75:119–128.

About the Author

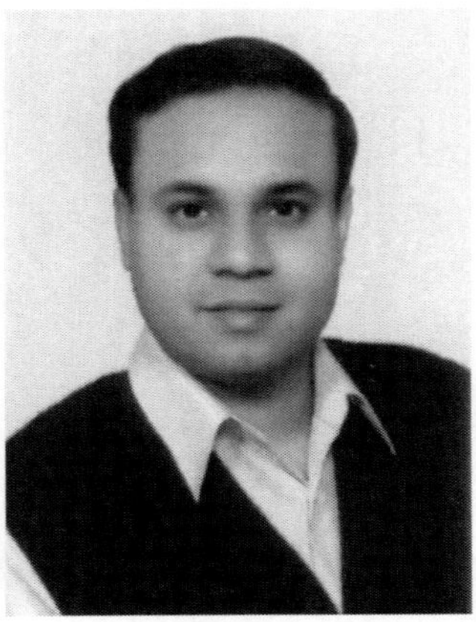

Dr. Devinder Preet Singh, BDS, MDS
Sr. Assistant Professor
Dept. of Orthodontics & Dentofacial Orthopedics
Dr. Harvansh Singh Judge Institute of Dental Sciences & Hospital
Panjab University, Chandigarh, India
Email: Ahluwalia147@gmail.com

Dr. Devinder Preet Singh is a specialist Orthodontist in the field of dentistry working as a Senior Assistant Professor in the Department Of Orthodontics & Dentofacial Orthopedics in Dr. Harvansh Singh Judge Institute of Dental Sciences & Hospital, Panjab University, Chandigarh, India for the last eight odd years. During his tenure he has been blessed with the opportunity to be able to carry out various research works in his field, many of which have been published in reputed international and national journals of his speciality. He is a Fellow Member of many reputed national and international bodies such as ICD,WFO, AAO, EOS, ADA, IOS, and IDA. He also had the opportunity to undertake important duties in the academic front such as Chairperson of Scientific Sessions/Member of Organising Committees / Sectional Secretary of the various conferences in the university. He has received numerous awards and recongnition for his work in his field such as the best paper award of Chandigarh Science Congress (CHASCON) 2012, PUTA Teacher's Day Award 2013, 'Profile Of The Month' Award for the month of May 2014 given by the IDA(Indian Dental Association) and the Highly Commendable and the Winner of the Specialist Of The Year (Orthodontist)for the year 2014 and 2015 respectively, organised by the FAMDENT India.

Index

A

adhesion, 46
adverse effects, 86
aesthetics, 20
alkaline phosphatase, 55
aluminum oxide, 52
alveolar ridge, 22, 41, 57, 112
alveolus, 78
anchorage, vii, 1, 5, 6, 7, 8, 9, 10, 11, 13, 14, 45, 48, 63, 65, 67, 69, 70, 71, 73, 74, 77, 81, 82, 86, 94, 97, 99, 117, 119, 120, 121, 124, 125
anchoring, 11
angulation, 94
ankylosis, 66, 68

B

basal lamina, 54
bicuspid, 97, 99, 100
bilateral, 64, 75, 124
bioactive materials, 39
biocompatibility, 31, 33, 38, 44, 45, 46, 51, 121, 123
biomaterials, 31
biomolecules, 35, 37
blood, 11, 15, 26, 55
blood pressure, 15
blood vessels, 11, 26, 55
bonding, 35, 37, 38, 39, 41, 43, 52, 54
bonds, 35, 39
bone(s), 3, 5, 6, 7, 8, 9, 10, 11, 12, 13, 14, 17, 18, 19, 21, 22, 23, 24, 25, 26, 27, 28, 29, 30, 32, 36, 38, 41, 42, 43, 44, 45, 46, 47, 48, 49, 51, 52, 54, 55, 56, 57, 59, 60, 64, 65, 67, 68, 72, 73, 75, 77, 78, 79, 80, 81, 83, 85, 86, 88, 91, 93, 94, 95, 96, 97, 99, 100, 103, 105, 109, 111, 113, 114, 115, 119, 120, 121, 122, 124
bone form, 13, 14, 43, 44, 56, 68, 85, 100
bone growth, 29, 41, 43
bone mass, 64
bone resorption, 41, 43, 52, 56, 111
bone volume, 11, 19, 21

C

CAD, 26, 122
calcification, 12, 111, 115
calcium, 38, 44, 52
calvaria, 121
CAM, 26, 122
canals, 111
capillary, 55
capsule, 3, 65, 119
carbon, 5, 31, 52, 54, 63, 119
cardiac risk factors, 15

cardiovascular disease(s), 15
ceramic(s), 29, 37, 39, 53
ceramic materials, 37
cortical bone, 12, 19, 72, 78, 92, 93, 94, 105
covalent bonding, 35
covering, 25, 80
crown(s), 3, 11, 13, 72, 83, 97, 99, 119
crystal structure, 34
crystallinity, 103
crystallization, 37
crystals, 38, 39
CT scan, 24
cuspids, 5, 63, 68

D

denaturation, 55
dental implants, 3, 7, 12, 19, 24, 27, 31, 32, 43, 119, 122, 123
dental offices, 18, 20, 21
dentin, 6
dentist, 18, 20, 21, 22, 24, 31, 77
dentistry, vii, 27, 31, 96, 122, 123
dentures, 3, 97, 122
discomfort, vii, 1, 41, 77, 97
distalization, vii, 1, 10, 13, 83, 84, 102, 125

E

extraction, 3, 5, 7, 8, 10, 11, 13, 43, 57, 69, 73, 94, 108, 120
extraction sites, 3, 5, 7, 11, 43

F

false teeth, 119
first molar, 5, 7, 8, 13, 18, 74, 86, 92, 103
fixation, 26, 41, 42, 101, 108, 114, 115, 124
force, 5, 6, 7, 8, 9, 11, 13, 20, 63, 64, 65, 67, 68, 69, 70, 71, 72, 83, 91, 96, 120, 121
fracture resistance, 31
fractures, 6, 103
fragments, 39, 109

G

gingival, 3, 54, 59, 60, 80, 104, 124

H

healing, vii, 1, 3, 6, 8, 10, 11, 13, 14, 16, 27, 51, 55, 56, 57, 58, 64, 67, 74, 77, 80, 85, 97, 105, 109, 110, 111, 114, 117
healing period, vii, 1, 6, 10, 11, 13, 14, 57, 58, 64, 77, 105, 117
hydroxide, 36
hydroxyapatite, 31, 81
hydroxylapatite, 123
hygiene, 55, 97

I

implant diameter, 42, 57
implant length, 42
implant placement, 21, 22, 56, 91, 92, 108
implant planning, 22
implantology, 28, 31, 122
implants, vii, 1, 3, 5, 6, 7, 8, 9, 10, 11, 12, 13, 14, 17, 18, 19, 20, 22, 24, 25, 26, 27, 28, 29, 30, 31, 32, 34, 35, 37, 41, 42, 43, 44, 45, 46, 51, 52, 54, 56, 57, 58, 59, 60, 61, 63, 64, 65, 67, 68, 69, 71, 73, 75, 77, 81, 91, 92, 93, 96, 97, 100, 103, 108, 110, 111, 112, 117, 119, 120, 121, 122, 123, 124, 125
incisor(s), 5, 7, 8, 10, 12, 13, 17, 60, 61, 66, 72, 74, 75, 78, 81, 86
intrusion(s), vii, 1, 8, 11, 13, 70, 71, 72, 121

L

light-cured composite, 97, 99
LINKOW, 1
local anesthesia, 78, 86, 97, 102
local anesthetic, 94

M

mandible, 13, 18, 19, 22, 24, 25, 26, 28, 49, 57, 64, 84, 85, 91, 92, 107, 108, 110, 111
marrow, 75, 115
materials, 3, 32, 34, 36, 44, 46, 51, 52
maxilla, 6, 10, 13, 22, 24, 25, 28, 49, 57, 68, 83, 91, 112, 114
maxillary expansion, vii, 1
maxillary incisors, 75
maxillary protraction, vii, 1, 124
maxillary sinus, 19
measurement(s), 5, 10, 12, 15, 22, 37
mechanical properties, 34, 38, 42
micro-implants, vii, 1, 92, 93, 96

N

nerve, 19, 85, 95, 108
niobium, 45, 54

O

oral cavity, 72, 106
Oral Implantology, 1, 122
oral implants, 1, 121
orthodontic anchorage, vii, 1, 5, 11, 13, 14, 63, 77, 97, 99, 119, 120, 124, 125
orthodontic implants, vii, 117
orthodontic treatment, 9, 10, 81, 86, 104
orthopedic, vii, 1, 9, 67, 120
ossification, 55, 111
osteoporosis, 47
osteotomy, 84, 89, 90, 112, 114
oxygen, 34, 36

P

pain, 97
palate, 7, 8, 10, 90, 95, 96, 100, 112
patient compliance, vii, 1, 117
patient discomfort, vii, 1, 41
peri-implant soft tissue, 11
periodontal, 7, 54, 64
periosteum, 109
porcelain crown, 3
premolars, 5, 7, 8, 9, 10, 11, 12, 60, 74, 83, 92, 103, 112

R

radiation, 21, 24, 58
reconstruction, 75, 103, 124
regeneration, 54, 55, 57, 58
rehabilitation, 17, 51, 123
reinforcement, 10, 117
repair, 103
root(s), 3, 7, 11, 12, 13, 17, 27, 28, 29, 31, 57, 64, 66, 68, 78, 91, 94, 96, 100, 101, 103, 121

S

scanning electron microscopy, 14
second molar, 7, 8, 83, 93, 100
Skeletal Anchorage System (SAS), vii, 1, 11, 13, 71
space closure, vii, 1, 7, 66, 70, 71
stability, 6, 7, 9, 10, 29, 32, 36, 43, 44, 46, 47, 65, 75, 101, 105
stabilization, 42, 57, 114, 115

T

tantalum, 31, 45, 54
techniques, vii, 19, 22, 24, 117
technological advancement, 1
technology, 24, 117
teeth, 3, 6, 7, 8, 10, 11, 12, 13, 17, 28, 54, 59, 60, 65, 66, 81, 82, 83, 86, 88, 91, 94, 100, 112, 119, 120, 124
temperature, 33, 35, 38, 48, 55, 56
tensile strength, 38
tension, 10, 11, 111
texture, 25, 29, 41, 42
therapy, 88, 122
third molar(s), 83

tissue, 6, 7, 13, 20, 22, 34, 38, 39, 41, 42, 43, 44, 45, 48, 51, 53, 54, 55, 56, 59, 60, 80, 81, 82, 89, 90, 91, 93, 94, 95, 96, 97, 111, 114, 115
titanium, 5, 6, 7, 8, 9, 10, 11, 12, 13, 27, 28, 31, 33, 34, 35, 36, 37, 43, 44, 45, 53, 54, 57, 63, 64, 66, 67, 68, 69, 72, 73, 80, 81, 91, 96, 97, 99, 100, 101, 103, 108, 111, 112, 120, 121, 123, 124
tooth, 3, 7, 11, 12, 13, 22, 57, 60, 65, 66, 81, 99, 108, 117, 119, 123
tooth implant, 3, 60, 123
TPA, 74, 75, 84
treatment, vii, 1, 3, 10, 12, 13, 15, 17, 24, 27, 32, 55, 59, 68, 72, 83, 86, 87, 88, 101, 121, 122, 123
treatment time, vii, 1, 88

V

vitallium implant, 3

X

x-rays, 91

Z

zirconia, 54
zygoma, 7, 68
zygomatic arch, 9